Math for Health Care Professionals

To my bride, Trisha. Thank you for being my best friend and partner.

To my three sons, Devin, Cody, and Lane. What a joy it is to see you three grow into young gentlemen.

To my parents, Kenneth and Mary Kennamer. Thank you for always being supportive in all I have done.

Math for Health Care Professionals

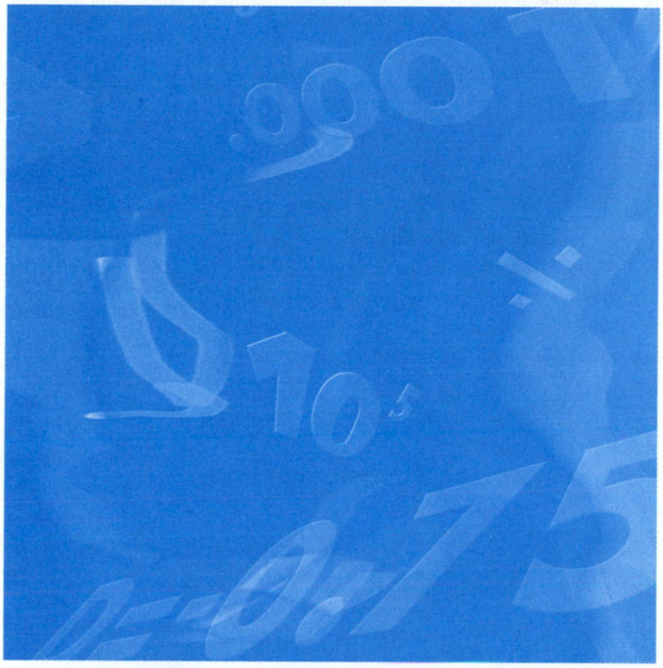

Mike Kennamer, EMT-P, MPA

Director of Adult Education and Skills Training Division
Northeast Alabama Community College
Rainsville, Alabama

THOMSON
DELMAR LEARNING

Australia Canada Mexico Singapore Spain United Kingdom United States

THOMSON

DELMAR LEARNING

Math for Health Care Professionals
by Mike Kennamer, EMT-P, MPA

Vice President, Health Care Business Unit:
William Brottmiller

Editorial Director:
Cathy L. Esperti

Acquisitions Editor:
Marah Bellegarde

Marketing Director:
Jennifer McAvey

Marketing Channel Manager:
Tamara Caruso

Senior Production Editor:
James Zayicek

Printed in the United States of America
1 2 3 4 5 XXX 09 08 07 06 05 04

For more information, contact Delmar Learning, 5 Maxwell Drive, Clifton Park, NY 12065. Or find us on the World Wide Web at http://www.delmarlearning.com

Library of Congress Cataloging-in-Publication Data

Kennamer, Mike.
Math for health care professionals / Mike Kennamer.
p. cm.
Includes bibliographical references and index.
ISBN 1-4018-5803-1
1. Medicine—Mathematics. I. Title.

R853.M3K46 2004
513'.027'61—dc22 2003068766

Notice to the Reader

CONTENTS

UNIT 2 BASIC PRINCIPLES

Chapter 5 Decimals / 55

Chapter 6 Fractions / 79

UNIT 3 APPLICATIONS

PREFACE

Math for Health Care Professionals provides a comprehensive mathematics text for students enrolled in, or interested in, any of the health care professions. Written at a level appropriate for both secondary and postsecondary students, *Math for Health Care Professionals* utilizes a unique competency-based approach in which instructors assess individual student abilities and prescribe learning activities that support the learning needs of each student. Whether used in the classroom or for independent study, the organization and structure of this book meets the learning needs of each student.

This book was written with both the instructor and student in mind. Instructors will enjoy the flexibility of selecting only the skills needed for each student from a cafeteria-style format. Instructors can also assign self-assessment pretests for each chapter to assess the knowledge and skills of each student. These assessments will help the instructor focus on the skills most needed by each student.

Students will enjoy the easy-to-read format and will benefit from thorough explanations of each concept presented. Of special interest to students will be the *Math in the Real World* features, where actual health care professionals share their thoughts on the importance of mathematics in everyday life. Other features important to students include self-assessment pretests, multiple opportunities for practice, and an excellent workbook that provides tremendous opportunities for directed practice.

ORGANIZATION

This text is organized in a logical fashion that helps the student move from understanding the basic principles to mastering more complicated operations. The student then utilizes these principles to perform application-level functions that require technical knowledge and critical thinking skills.

Unit 1 describes the importance of mathematics as a function of health care professionals. Unit 2 clearly explains the skills that are vitally important for health care professionals, and Unit 3 puts these skills into action with actual health care applications. Unit 4 provides students with a collection of resources that will be helpful throughout their careers.

FEATURES

- **Learning objectives** for each chapter are clear and measurable.
- **Key terms** listed at the beginning of each chapter are shown as bold in the text and defined both in the chapter and in the glossary.
- **Math in the Real World** is a feature of each chapter that highlights a health care professional explaining the importance of mathematical skills for health care professionals.
- A **Self-Assessment Pretest** allows the student to assess competency in each of the skills covered by the chapter learning objectives.
- **Skill Sharpener exercises** are offered after each section to give the student additional practice on each skill.
- **Review and Reflect** provides thought-provoking questions to exercise critical thinking skills.
- **Answers** to selected Self-Assessment Pretests, Skill Sharpener exercises, and Review and Reflect questions appear at the back of the book.

ALSO AVAILABLE

For the Student

Workbook to Accompany Math for Health Care Professionals

Order number 1-4018-9179-9

The workbook provides hundreds of questions for practice and mastery of each of the objectives included in the book.

Math for Health Care Professionals Quick Review

Order number 1-4018-8005-3

This quick review guide is intended for those with prior demonstrated knowledge of basic mathematical principles. It serves as review and, accordingly, does not include the self-assessment pretests found in the core book. It is ideal for those who need a quick refresher of mathematical concepts.

For the Instructor

Instructor's Manual to Accompany Math for Health Care Professionals

Order number 1-4018-9113-6

This handy instructor resource includes answers to all the problems in the book, workbook, and quick review guide. It provides assessment and evaluation tools that will help instructors direct students to areas that require the most attention.

ABOUT THE AUTHOR

Mike Kennamer is a graduate of the paramedic program at Gadsden State Community College in Gadsden, Alabama. He holds a B.S. in public safety administration from Athens State University in Athens, Alabama and an M.P.A. from Jacksonville State University in Jacksonville, Alabama. He is currently enrolled in the doctoral program in higher education administration at the University of Alabama in Tuscaloosa.

Mr. Kennamer currently serves as director of the Adult Education and Skills Training Division at Northeast Alabama Community College in Rainsville, where he oversees a number of vocational programs including paramedic, pharmacy technician, medical assistant, nursing assistant, and home health aide. He is the author of *Basic Infection Control for Health Care Providers, Instructor Manual to Accompany Delmar Learning's Basic Core Skills for Nursing Assistants, Delmar's Basic Life Support Video Series,* and *Delmar's Advanced Life Support Video Series,* and served as scriptwriter for *Delmar Learning's Basic Core Skills for Nursing Assistants.*

ACKNOWLEDGMENTS

The author wishes to thank the following reviewers who provided valuable input on the content and structure of this book.

Linda Taylor, MT
MLT Instructor
Apollo College
Phoenix, AZ

Donna Powers, RNC, BSN
Former Instructor
Health Occupations Education
Bound Brook, NJ

Elizabeth McPeak, RN
Instructor
Southeast Regional Occupational Program and North Orange County Regional Occupational Program
Lakewood, CA

Cindy Pavel, MPA, BA, BS, MT, CMT
Department Coordinator
School of Health Professions
Davenport University
Granger, IN

Special thanks to the following companies for providing medication labels.

Eli Lilly & Company
Keflex

Endo Pharmaceuticals
Percocet

Hoechst-Roussel Pharmaceuticals
Lasix

Luitpold Pharmaceuticals
Furosemide Injection

Merck & Company, Inc.
Comvax
M-M-R II
Mevacor
Singulair

Pharmacia Corporation
Celebrex

SmithKline Beecham
Infanrix

The author also wishes to recognize the valuable contributions of those individuals who participated the *Math in the Real World* features. Their experience and expertise is of tremendous value to the students who will learn from these professionals. Those who participated include:

Laurie A. Romig, M.D., F.A.C.E.P.
Medical Director
Pinellas County EMS
Pinellas County, Florida

Barbara Hammond
Radiology Assistant
St. Francis Medical Center
Grand Island, Nebraska

Mike Harper, CRNA, JD
Anesthetist
Gadsden Regional Medical Center
Gadsden, Alabama

Robert Lewis, RPh
Pharmacist
Bi-Lo Pharmacy
Trenton, Georgia

Roger G. Wootten, AAS, EMT-P
EMS Instructional Coordinator
Northeast Alabama Community College
Rainsville, Alabama
and
Paramedic
DeKalb Ambulance Service
Fort Payne, Alabama

Others who contributed to this book by providing photos or by being photographed include:

Laura H. Alexander – photographer (Unit Three title page)

Barbara Hammond – subject of photo (Unit Two title page)

Joyce Mitchell – subject of photo (Unit Three title page)

Carmen Steckline – subject of photo (Unit Two title page)

As always, the Delmar Learning team was wonderful to work with. This project was signed by Acquisitions Editor Sherry Gomoll. Thanks Sherry, for always going the extra mile for your authors. Your hard work and commitment to producing the best possible product is much appreciated.

Initial work was handled through Sherry Gomoll and her Editorial Assistant, Jennifer Conklin. Thanks to Jennifer for fielding all my questions and for helping me to convert the *Math in the Real World* feature from concept to reality.

When Sherry was promoted to Director of Career Education, this project was driven by the team of Marah Bellegarde, Acquisitions Editor; Erin Adams, Editorial Assistant; and Senior Production Editor, Jim Zayicek. Marah willingly listened to my input and concerns and kept an open mind when considering my suggestions. Erin was very helpful with early edits and formatting advice and did her best to keep me on track. Jim worked behind the scenes to make sure the project stayed on track and that each aspect of production went smoothly.

Thanks is also due to Judi Orozco of TDB Publishing Services, who provided the talent and skill that turned reams of computer-generated manuscript and my doodled notes into the attractive book you are now reading.

And of course, thanks are always due to my family, who continue to support and encourage me through the completion of each project I tackle. I could not ask for a better partner in this business, and in life, than my wife, Trisha. Our three sons, Devin, Cody, and Lane, are always a source of inspiration and often a much needed diversion from writing.

FEEDBACK

The author is interested in hearing from anyone who would like to offer suggestions or constructive criticism for future editions of this book. Also, health care professionals who are interested in participating in the *Math in the Real World* segment in future editions should contact the author through Delmar Learning or directly by email at kennamerm@nacc.edu.

TO THE READER

Welcome to the exciting and rewarding field of health care. Regardless of the health care profession you pursue, be assured that your chosen profession will be one that impacts the lives of other people on a daily basis. Your work as a health care professional will be valuable, and your studies in preparing for that career are equally important.

This book is a tool to help you assure success in your chosen field of study. The skills and abilities you learn through this book include some that you will continue to use in daily life. Please take the time necessary for study to ensure that you have mastered each of the objectives presented.

STUDY TIPS

You may find that this textbook is set up differently from others you may have used. Most books present a list of learning objectives and then cover each of the objectives somewhere within the chapter. This book is a little different in that it lists a learning objective, then immediately discusses that objective.

It is important to understand the value of objectives. Objectives are much like goals. In other words, each learning objective listed in this book is like a learning goal. Perhaps you can approach your study with that concept in mind. As you progress to each learning objective, make mastering the knowledge, skill, or ability in that objective your goal for that period in time. Work on that objective until you achieve mastery, then progress to the next objective.

This book is also set up in such a way that your instructor may tell you to skip one or more objectives. This may be because your instructor has evidence that you have already mastered a specific objective or set of objectives or because a specific objective or group of objectives do not relate to your field of study. Please understand that this represents sound educational theory but realize that you may, if necessary, work on objectives that are not assigned if you believe you need additional work in a particular area.

The accompanying workbook is very helpful in this regard and offers dozens of questions for you to practice. Please consider using this resource for additional practice that will lead to mastery of your mathematical skills.

CALCULATORS

Calculators are a valuable tool and are used regularly in health care. However, a good health care professional should understand how to calculate any problem in this book without the aid of a calculator. If your instructor allows you to use a calculator, utilize it as a valuable tool, but also practice working some of the problems without a calculator so that you will understand how to solve problems when a calculator is not available.

Many of you will take certification and/or licensure exams as you progress in your health care career. Keep in mind that many of the certification and licensing agencies do not allow the use of a calculator during testing. Learn the requirements for the exam(s) that you will take and practice accordingly.

CONCLUSION

I hope that you find as much enjoyment during your career as a health care professional as I have had as a field paramedic and a paramedic instructor. Whatever you decide to do—whether you enter a career in health care or not—do what you enjoy.

Your patients will be able to tell if you really enjoy your work. Your attitude will reflect on the care you provide and how you interact with co-workers, your patients' families, and others you come in contact with. Let your patients know you care and that you are there to give them the best possible care.

UNIT

1

Introduction

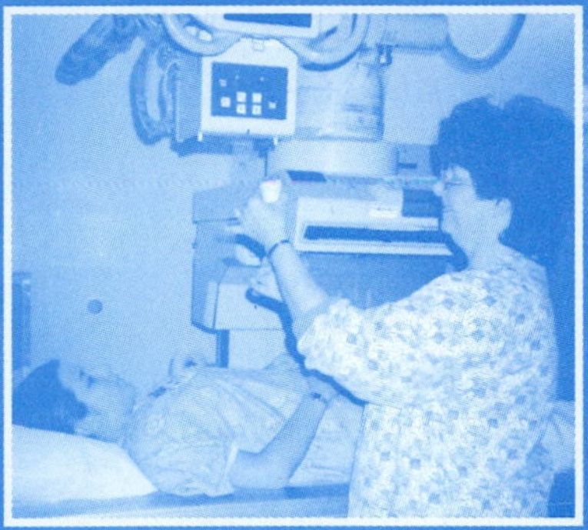

This unit provides evidence that mathematics is a valuable skill used by health care professionals on a daily basis. As a vital health care tool, mathematics will help the health care professional provide the best care to patients.

Each health care field holds its own set of requirements and skill competencies. However, every health care discipline requires competency (at varied levels) in math skills. A strong foundation in mathematics is essential to success in the health care profession.

CHAPTER 1

Math As a Health Care Function

LEARNING **OBJECTIVES**

After completing this chapter, the reader will be able to:

- **1.1** List at least three ways math is used in everyday life.
- **1.2** Recognize mathematics as a vital health care skill.
- **1.3** List at least three ways math is used in different health care disciplines.

KEY **TERMS**

- hard skills
- soft skills

MATH IN THE REAL WORLD

"Learning to do word problems as a kid is one of the most useful things you'll ever do. It's one of the first things you learn that ends up imitating everyday math skills that everyone needs! They train your brain to think in an organized, problem-solving way."

Laurie A. Romig, MD, FACEP

SELF-ASSESSMENT **PRETEST**

1. List three ways you use math in everyday life.

2. Discuss the importance of math in your health care discipline.

INTRODUCTION

Every day, health care providers utilize the knowledge, skills, and abilities that come together as a skill set needed for a particular occupation. Among these skills are **hard skills**, like starting intravenous lines and taking an x-ray, as well as **soft skills**, like communicating with patients and their family members and reading (Figure 1-1). Both types of skills are vitally important to success in a health care career. However, students should have a firm foundation of soft skills upon which to build their hard skills, or technical expertise.

One of the most vital soft skills involves mathematics, which health care providers use daily in both their personal and professional lives. Think of all the ways numbers and mathematics are used on a daily basis. Could you function for even one day without math and numbers?

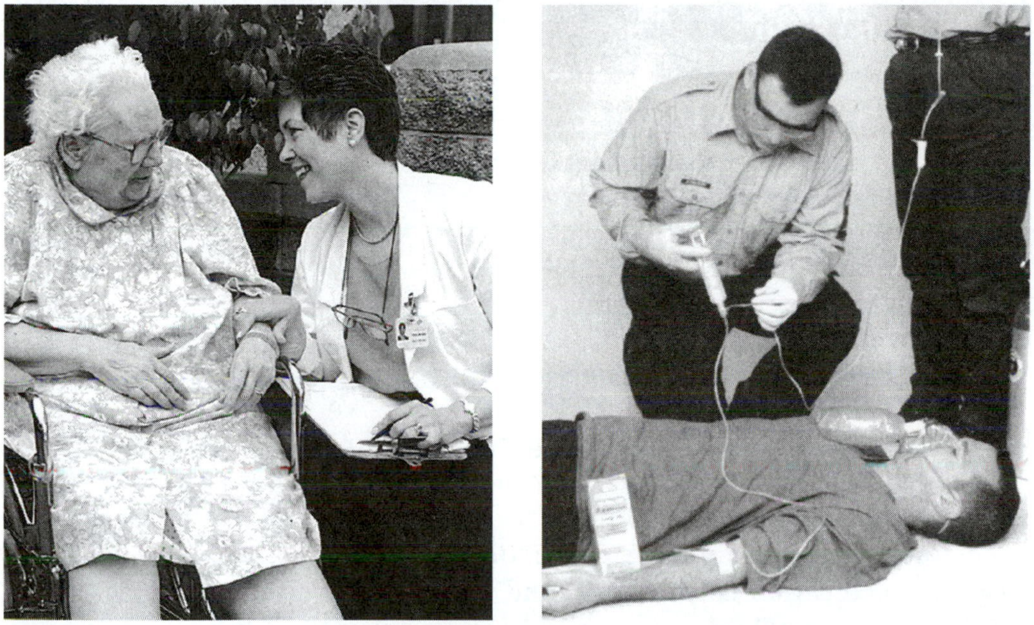

FIGURE 1-1 Health care professionals must possess both soft skills like reading, math, and communication skills and hard skills specifically related to their profession.

Objective

1.1 List at least three ways math is used in everyday life.

People from all walks of life utilize mathematics every day in a variety of ways. When you wake up to an alarm clock, a numerical system is telling you what time it is. To make coffee in the morning, you use proportions to mix the correct amount of coffee for the amount of water used. When driving to work, you may use fractions to check to see if you need gas in your car. You pay for your lunch with money, which is measured using decimals. The sales tax you pay is figured as a percentage, and added to your total. The soft drink you purchase may be packaged in a bottle measured in liters. As illustrated in Figure 1-2, math, as you may have determined by now, is an important part of your everyday life.

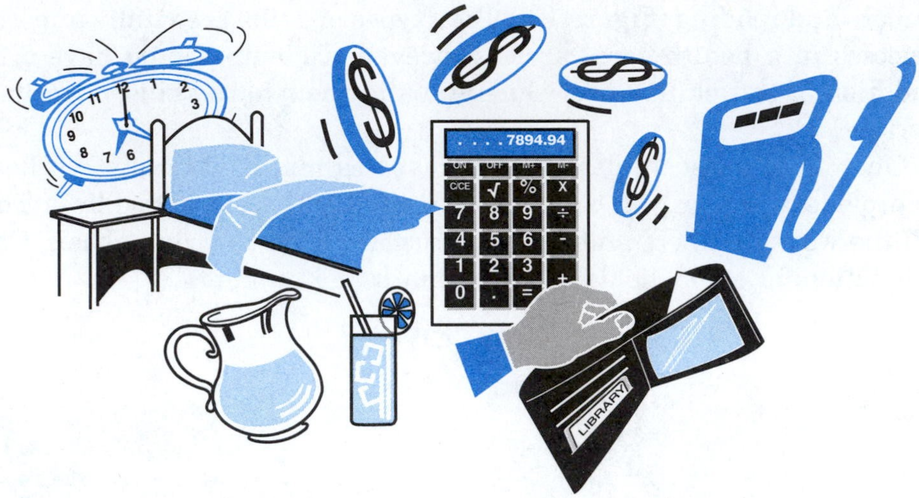

FIGURE 1-2 Just a few of the ways we use math in everyday life.

Objective

1.2 Recognize mathematics as a vital health care skill.

Health care providers use math as part of daily job skills. Many of the skills health care providers perform depend on mathematical calculations for accuracy. Health care providers utilize mathematical skills like proportions and fractions when figuring medication dosages. Decimals are commonly used in medication calculations, and percents are used for many things, from intravenous fluid concentrations to oxygen administration.

Understanding the importance of math is vital to success in any health care discipline. While different disciplines require varied levels of mathematical knowledge, health care providers at any level need a firm foundation of mathematics that, coupled with other basic soft skills like written and oral communication, reading, and locating information, will help them to be successful.

Objective

1.3 List at least three ways math is used in different health care disciplines.

Regardless of what health care discipline you choose, you will find that math is an important skill. Figure 1-3 illustrates a variety of mathematical applications used by people in different health care fields.

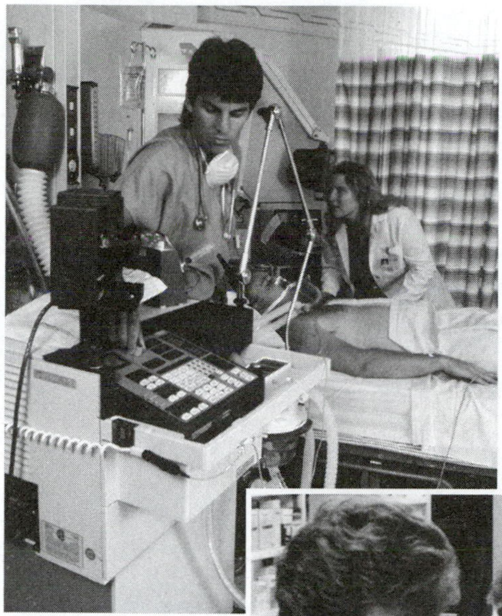

Respiratory Therapist

- Setting up ventilators
- Calculating medication dosages
- Analyzing arterial blood gas results

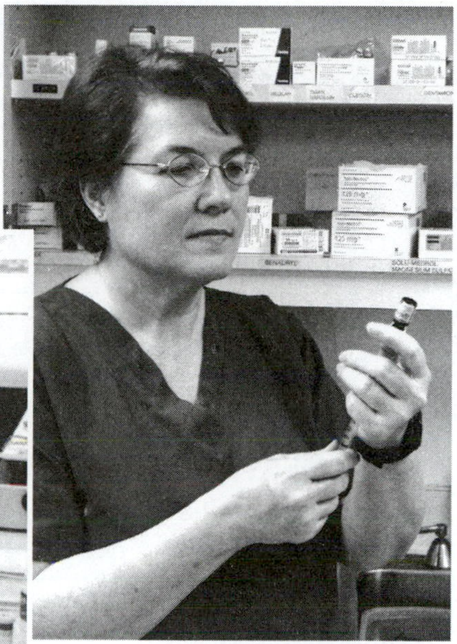

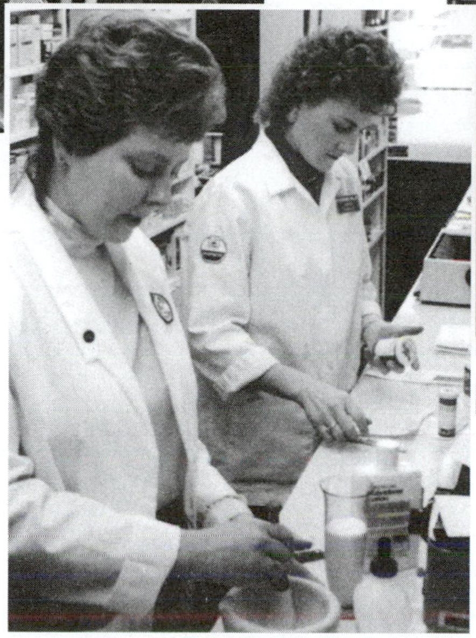

Registered Nurse

- Calculating medication dosages
- Entering data into computers
- Explaining to patients how much medication to take by converting to household measurements

Pharmacist

- Reading prescriptions
- Converting from one system to another
- Explaining dosages to patients

FIGURE 1-3 Health care professionals use math every day in their jobs.

CONCLUSION

Throughout history, mathematics and numbers have been an important part of everyday life. Today we live in a world where evidence of the importance of math is all around us. Computers, for instance, operate on a numerical system called the binary system, which consists of only two digits—0 and 1.

A strong foundation of mathematical skills is key to success in health care, regardless of the health care discipline you plan to enter. Ratios and proportions, fractions, decimals, and percents are all considered vital in any health care profession.

REVIEW AND REFLECT

1. Other than mathematics, what are some soft skills that a health care professional should have?

2. What are some of the soft skills that everyone in the work force should have?

3. Which mathematical operations do you believe will be most helpful in your chosen field of study?

4. List at least three hard skills that you will learn in your program of study.

5. Do you enjoy math? Why or why not?

UNIT 2

Basic Principles

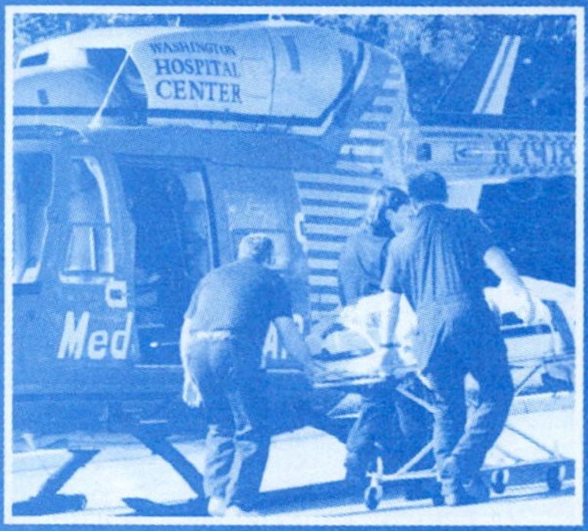

This unit provides a stable foundation of mathematical skills upon which the student may build. Each chapter features a self-assessment pretest that can be used to better understand individual strengths and identify areas where further study and practice are needed.

A thorough understanding of the principles discussed in this unit will help in the successful application of these principles when presented in Unit 3 and in actual practice.

CHAPTER 2

Numerical Systems

LEARNING OBJECTIVES

After completing this chapter, the reader will be able to:

- **2.1** List the common numerical systems in use today.
- **2.2** Convert Roman numerals to Hindu-Arabic numerals.
- **2.3** Convert Hindu-Arabic numerals to Roman numerals.

KEY TERMS

- Hindu-Arabic system
- numerical system
- Roman numerals

MATH IN THE REAL WORLD

"In the practice of pharmacy, we see Roman numerals used a lot in prescription writing. Mainly they are used to denote the number of units in the dosage of a medication. An illustration would be, "ii tabs tid," which would mean "take 2 tablets three times daily."

Robert Lewis, Registered Pharmacist

SELF-ASSESSMENT **PRETEST**

Convert the following Roman numerals to Arabic.

1. IV ______
2. XII ______
3. MCLIV ______
4. V ______
5. VIII ______
6. XXXVI ______
7. XIX ______
8. CXC ______
9. MCMLXXXIII ______
10. MCMLXV ______

Convert the following Arabic numerals to Roman.

1. 2,003 ______
2. 14 ______
3. 98 ______
4. 3,456 ______
5. 231 ______
6. 798 ______
7. 465 ______
8. 2 ______
9. 72 ______
10. 112 ______

INTRODUCTION

Numerical systems, or organized systems for counting, are as old as civilization itself. For centuries, people have used numbers to trade with each other and to keep records. Whether they made scratch marks on a rock, or perhaps used pebbles or their fingers to count, people have used numbers throughout history.

Objective

2.1 List the common numerical systems in use today.

We commonly use the **Hindu-Arabic system** of numbers, though **Roman numerals** are still sometimes used. Although health care professionals are not frequently called upon to use Roman numerals, you should be able to convert from Roman to Hindu-Arabic numbers.

ROMAN NUMERALS

Almost 3,000 years ago, the people of ancient Rome developed a numerical system that is still used today, but only on a limited basis. This system has evolved from tick marks on a rock or the ground (as shown in Figure 2-1) into the additive system it is today. Numbers are read by adding and subtracting a series of symbols. The symbols used include the following:

I = 1	C = 100
V = 5	D = 500
X = 10	M = 1,000
L = 50	

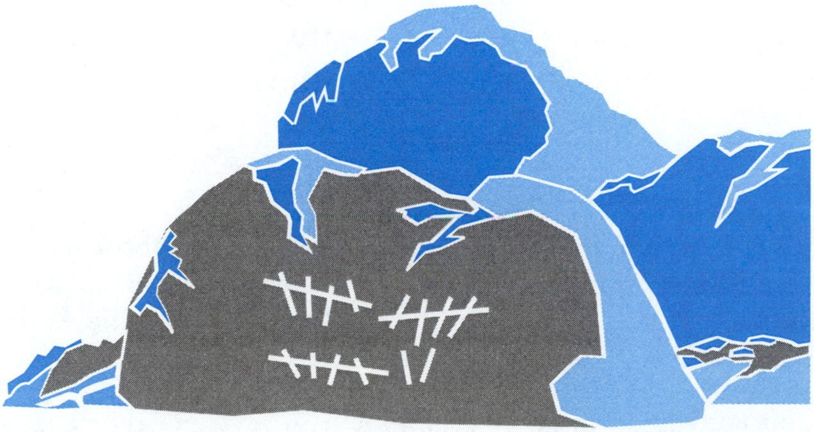

FIGURE 2-1 Roman numerals are believed to have evolved from something as simple as tick marks on a rock.

These symbols are combined to create any number. If a symbol for a lower number is placed before another symbol, the lower symbol is subtracted from the other. If the lower symbol follows the larger symbol, the symbols should be added. For example, by placing the I in front of the V, we subtract 1 from 5. By placing the I after the V, we must add 1 to the 5.

I is equal to 1	I
II is equal to 2	I + I
III is equal to 3	I + I + I
IV is equal to 4	V – I
V is equal to 5	V
VI is equal to 6	V + I
VII is equal to 7	V + I + I
VIII is equal to 8	V + I + I + I
IX is equal to 9	X – I
X is equal to 10	X

The same principles apply to larger numbers as illustrated in the following examples.

Example

X + X + V + I + I = XXVII

10 + 10 + 5 + 1 + 1 = 27

Example

MCMXXXIV

M + (M – C) + X + X + X + (V – I)

1000 + (1000 – 100) + 10 + 10 + 10 + (5 – 1)

1000 + 900 + 10 + 10 + 10 + 4 = 1934

HINDU-ARABIC NUMBERS

The numerical system ordinarily used in the United States is called the *Hindu-Arabic system*. This system was developed around 600 A.D. in India by the Hindus and was brought to the Western world by the Arabs about one hundred years later. Today, we refer to this system as Hindu-Arabic or simply Arabic.

This system is based on the digits 0, 1, 2, 3, 4, 5, 6, 7, 8, and 9. By combining these digits, any number can be represented.

Objective

2.2 Convert Roman numerals to Hindu-Arabic numerals.

To convert Roman numerals to Hindu-Arabic numbers, convert the Roman symbols to Hindu-Arabic symbols and add or subtract as previously described. For example, to convert XVII to Hindu-Arabic numbers, first convert each of the Roman numerals to Hindu-Arabic as follows:

X = 10	
V = 5	
I = 1	
I = 1	

Then add these numbers to find the sum of 17.

$10 + 5 + 1 + 1 = 17$

SKILL SHARPENER

Convert the following Roman numerals to Hindu-Arabic numerals.

1. XXVI ______
2. DCLI ______
3. DCI ______
4. MCL ______
5. CXXXVIII ______
6. MCMLXV ______
7. MM ______
8. MMMDXL ______
9. XXIV ______
10. DCLX ______

Objective

2.3 Convert Hindu-Arabic numerals to Roman numerals.

Convert Hindu-Arabic numerals to Roman numerals by using the same principles as converting Roman to Hindu-Arabic. For example, to convert the Hindu-Arabic number 129 to Roman numerals, first select the largest Roman numeral that equals a portion of this number.

C = 100

Subtract this number from the original number.

129 − 100 = 29

Now find the largest number that equals a portion of this number.

X = 10

Since X is the largest Roman numeral you can use, decide how many Xs are needed by dividing 10 into 29. The 10 will go into 29 twice; therefore, place two Xs to the right of the C.

CXX = 120

Subtract this number from the original number.

129 − 120 = 9

Since 9 can be represented as IX, add this to the right of the Roman numeral being created.

CXXIX = 129

SKILL SHARPENER

Convert the following Hindu-Arabic numerals to Roman numerals.

1. 145 ____________________

2. 3,420 ____________________

3. 312 ____________________

4. 453 ____________________

5. 1,394 ______________________

6. 1,250 ______________________

7. 38 ______________________

8. 365 ______________________

9. 3,217 ______________________

10. 333 ______________________

CONCLUSION

Roman numerals are not commonly used in today's health care system. However, it is important that health care professionals know how to convert between Roman and Hindu-Arabic systems if necessary. The remainder of this book will focus on the Hindu-Arabic system.

REVIEW AND REFLECT

1. Are there numerical systems other than those discussed in this chapter?

____

____

____

____

____

2. Other than medicine and health care, in what ways are Roman numerals used?

____

____

____

____

____

3. Why is the Roman number system referred to as an additive system?

4. In approximately what year did the Romans develop their numerical system?

5. When was the Hindu-Arabic system brought to the Western world?

CHAPTER 3

Measurement Systems

LEARNING **OBJECTIVES**

After completing this chapter, the reader will be able to:

- **3.1** List systems of measurement commonly utilized in the health care industry.
- **3.2** List and define key components of the apothecary system.
- **3.3** List and define key components of the household system.
- **3.4** List and define key components of the metric system.

KEY **TERMS**

- apothecary system
- English system
- household system
- metric system

MATH IN THE REAL WORLD

"I commonly interact with people who routinely do use the metric system, and those who don't. I need to be able to convert numbers into the format that means the most to the individual. Telling a parent how many teaspoons or milliliters or "mLs" of a medicine to give is a great example. For example, I want the parent to give the child 150 mg of a liquid medication that comes in a concentration of 200 mg/mL. How many mL should the parent give the child? How do you convert that to teaspoons or tablespoons?"

Laurie A. Romig, MD, FACEP

"Though apothecary measurements are not often seen today, we must be familiar with them so that when we are called upon to give 1/150 grain nitroglycerine, we will be able to understand that the order refers to the 0.4 mg tablets that we carry."

Roger G. Wootten, AAS, NREMT-Paramedic

SELF-ASSESSMENT **PRETEST**

Match the following units of measure with the appropriate system by placing A, B, or C in the blanks.

A	Apothecary system
B	Household system
C	Metric system

______ **1.** minim

______ **2.** gram

______ **3.** tablespoon

______ **4.** hectoliter

______ **5.** fluidounce

______ **6.** cup

______ **7.** fluidram

______ **8.** teaspoon

______ **9.** grain

______ **10.** pint

INTRODUCTION

Health care providers utilize a variety of measurement systems, and combinations of those systems, in carrying out tasks such as medication administration, weighing and measuring patients, and measuring intake and output. As a health care provider, you will be called upon to use these measurement systems and to convert between systems.

Health care and medicine are as old as civilization itself. Ancient parchments tell of caring for the sick and injured. The measurement systems in use today include a combination of ancient systems, like the apothecary and household systems, and the more modern metric system. Tradition has played a part in the hodgepodge of systems utilized today.

This chapter discusses each of the three measurement systems in use today. While some are used far more than others, it is important to understand the relationships of measurements within each system and how each system relates to each of the others. Conversions between systems will be covered in Chapter 9.

Objective

3.1 List systems of measurement commonly utilized in the health care industry.

Three systems of measurement are commonly utilized in the health care industry. They include the:

- apothecary system.
- household system.
- metric system.

Though the **apothecary system** is not common today, it is still used in some situations and health care professionals should be equipped to convert between this and other systems. Measurements like dram, fluidram, and minim are examples of apothecary system measures.

It is important to be able to convert to the **household system** so that the health care professional can assist patients with converting from metric and apothecary systems to more familiar measures. The household system is also called the **English system** because it originated in England. Examples of household system measurements include teaspoon, tablespoon, cup, and glass.

Though the **metric system** is used on a limited basis in the United States, it is the system most used for medication administration. Milliliters, milligrams, grams, liters, and cubic centimeters are metric system measurements utilized in the health care profession. Each of these systems will be discussed further within this chapter.

Objective

3.2 List and define key components of the apothecary system.

The apothecary system is an old English system of weight in which whole numbers are represented by Roman numerals, and normal fractions are used to express fractional parts. One-half is sometimes expressed as "ss." This system is frequently utilized for measuring medication dosages using weight or volume.

APOTHECARY SYSTEM OF WEIGHT

The apothecary system of weight utilizes the terms and symbols illustrated in Figure 3-1. It is worth noting that in this system, 480 grains equals one ounce and 12 ounces equals one pound. In contrast, in the household system, 16 ounces equals one pound.

Term	Abbreviation or Symbol
dram	dr or ʒ
grain	gr
ounce	oz or ℥
pound	lb

FIGURE 3-1 Apothecary units of weight

Therefore, you can expect to see medication orders using the apothecary system written as follows:

gr. vii	(7 grains)
℥ iii	(3 ounces)
ʒ ss	(1/2 dram)

SKILL SHARPENER

Write each of the following measurements using apothecary system symbols.

1. 3 grains ____________

2. $\frac{2}{3}$ dram ____________

3. 8 ounces ____________

4. 4 pounds ____________

5. $\frac{1}{200}$ of a grain ______________________

6. $\frac{1}{2}$ dram ______________________

7. 3 ounces ______________________

8. 2 pounds ______________________

9. 2 pounds and 11 ounces ______________________

10. $\frac{1}{2}$ grain ______________________

APOTHECARY SYSTEM OF VOLUME

The apothecary system of volume utilizes the terms illustrated in Figure 3-2. Though rarely used in today's health care professions, you should be able to convert between these and other systems.

Term	Abbreviation or Symbol
fluidounce	floz
fluidram	fldr or fl ʒ
gallon	gal
minim	m or ♍
pint	pt
quart	qt

FIGURE 3-2 Apothecary units of liquid volume

SKILL SHARPENER

Write each of the following measurements using apothecary system symbols.

1. 4 minims ______________________

2. 1 fluidram ______________________

3. 3 fluidounces ______________________

4. $\frac{1}{2}$ pint ______________________

5. 2 quarts ______________________

6. 3 gallons ______________________

7. 2 minims ______________________

8. 8 fluidounces ______________________

9. 5 fluidrams ________________

10. $2\frac{1}{2}$ gallons ________________

Objective

3.3 List and define key components of the household system.

The household system of measurement is primarily used when prescribing medication to be taken at home. Though the household system is not as accurate as other systems of measurement, health care providers must be familiar with it to instruct patients in taking correct dosages of their medications at home. Key components of the household system are listed in Figure 3-3.

Term	Abbreviation
drop	gtt
teaspoon	t or tsp
tablespoon	T or tbsp
teacup (6 oz)	tcp
cup or glass (8 oz)	C
pint	pt
quart	qt
gallon	gal
ounce	oz

FIGURE 3-3 Household units of measure

Objective

3.4 List and define key components of the metric system.

The metric system is used for many types of measurements in health care. Based on multiples of ten, metric measurements use whole numbers and decimals, rather than fractions, to express fractional parts.

METRIC PREFIXES AND SYMBOLS

The metric system uses prefixes that may be added to units of measure to alter their value. For instance, the prefix kilo-, meaning thousand, may be added to meter to signify one thousand meters. In similar fashion, the prefix

Unit	Value	Symbol
mega-	1,000,000	M
kilo-	1,000	k
hecto-	100	h
deka-	10	da
base	1	
deci-	0.1 or 1/10	d
centi-	0.01 or 1/100	c
milli-	0.001 or 1/1000	m
micro-	0.000001 or 1/1,000,000	µ or mc

FIGURE 3-4 Metric prefixes

milli-, meaning thousandth, may be added to meter to signify one thousandth of a meter. Other metric prefixes and their symbols are shown in Figure 3-4.

SKILL SHARPENER

Write the value that the following prefixes signify.

1. deci- ________________

2. deka- ________________

3. kilo- ________________

4. micro- ________________

5. milli- ________________

6. hecto- ________________

7. centi- ________________

METRIC UNITS OF MEASURE

Metric measurements are utilized by health care providers to measure weight, length, and volume (Figure 3-5). Whether measuring great distances using kilometers or making miniscule measurements using micrometers, the base unit of measure is the same—the meter. Similarly,

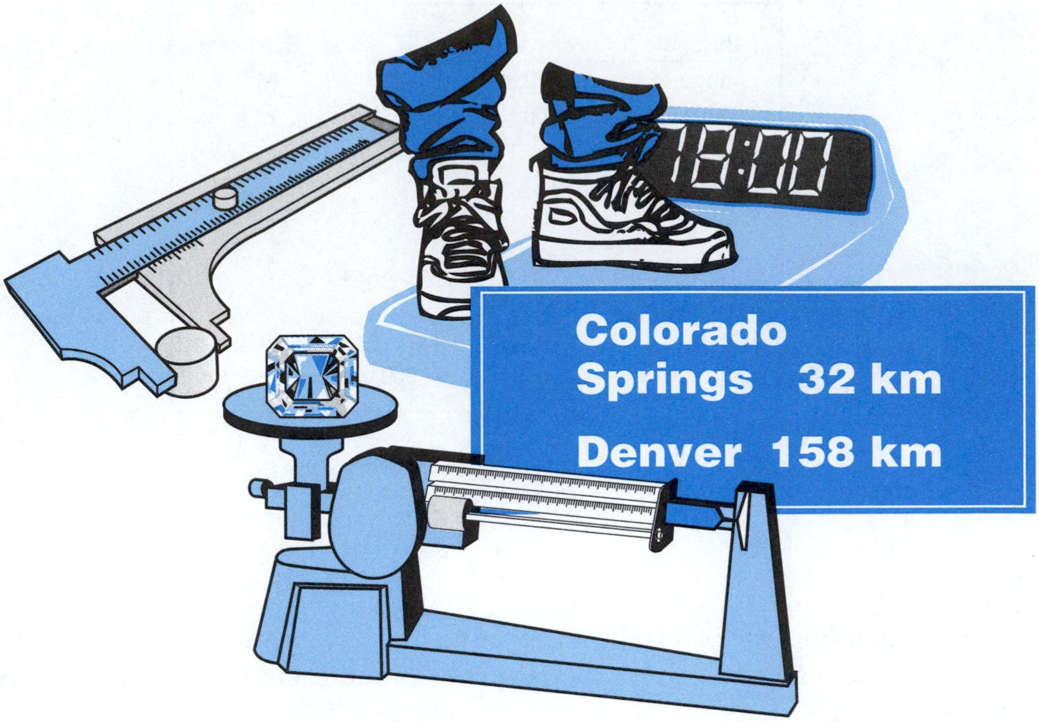

FIGURE 3-5 Though not widely embraced in the United States, the metric system is used for certain purposes, including health care and medicine.

the liter is the base unit of measure for volume, and gram is the base unit of measurement for weight.

SKILL SHARPENER

For each of the following, note whether the term is used to measure volume, weight, or length and whether the unit listed is a multiple of the base (ten, hundred, or thousand) or a fractional component (tenth, hundredth, thousandth, millionth) of the base.

	Measure of	Multiple or Fractional
1. millimeter	____________	______________________
2. deciliter	____________	______________________
3. hectometer	____________	______________________

4. milliliter ____________ ________________________

5. milligram ____________ ________________________

6. dekaliter ____________ ________________________

7. microliter ____________ ________________________

8. hectogram ____________ ________________________

9. kilogram ____________ ________________________

10. centimeter ____________ ________________________

CONCLUSION

It is important for the health care provider to understand the relationships between each of the measurement systems. Though the apothecary system is rarely used today, it is sometimes seen. The ability to understand each system and its relationship to other systems, as well as how measurements within a single system relate, is important in the overall care of patients.

REVIEW AND REFLECT

1. Why do you suppose there is not just one system of measurement?

____

____

____

____

____

2. The metric system is based on multiples of ________________________.

3. Which measurement system do you think is the most precise? Why?

____

____

____

____

____

4. Which measurement system are you the most comfortable with? Why?

____

____

____

____

____

5. Which measurement system do you believe to be the best suited to medical care? Why?

____

____

____

____

____

CHAPTER

4

Whole Number Review

LEARNING OBJECTIVES

After completing this chapter, the reader will be able to:

- 4.1 Define whole number.
- 4.2 Explain place value of whole numbers.
- 4.3 Compare whole numbers.
- 4.4 Order whole numbers.
- 4.5 Round whole numbers.
- 4.6 Add whole numbers.
- 4.7 Subtract whole numbers.
- 4.8 Multiply whole numbers.
- 4.9 Divide whole numbers.
- 4.10 Average whole numbers.

MATH IN THE REAL WORLD

"I cannot overestimate the importance of estimation in my everyday life. Because I understand the principle that multiplication is really just another form of addition, and division is just another form of subtraction, I can quickly come up with pretty good estimates of a calculation before anybody else can drag out a calculator!"

Laurie A. Romig, MD, FACEP

KEY TERMS

- addend
- average
- borrow
- difference
- dividend
- divisor
- factor
- mean
- minuend
- multiplicand
- multiplier
- place value
- product
- quotient
- remainder
- subtrahend
- sum
- whole number

SELF-ASSESSMENT **PRETEST**

Circle the digit found in the one's place.

1. 23

2. 543

3. 78

4. 93

5. 1

6. 34

7. 998

8. 3,292

9. 56,732

10. 750

Circle the digit found in the ten's place.

11. 124

12. 376

13. 89,977

14. 4,965

15. 324

16. 10,922

17. 300

18. 12

19. 13,545

20. 10

Circle the digit found in the hundred's place.

21. 123

22. 9,878

23. 13,243

24. 45,878

25. 990

26. 765

27. 78,900

28. 200

29. 43,342

30. 65,400

Circle the digit in the thousand's place.

31. 12,390

32. 78,980

33. 32,534

34. 1,200

35. 9,878

36. 45,000

37. 123,000

38. 454,302

39. 500,954

40. 231,493

Circle the digit in the ten thousand's place.

41. 14,390

42. 54,322

43. 299,987

44. 298,773

45. 12,098

46. 34,094

47. 150,900

48. 54,000

49. 893,204

50. 434,000

Circle the digit found in the hundred thousand's place.

51. 756,321

52. 1,235,434

53. 34,343,665

54. 1,200,900

55. 2,987,655

56. 45,443,345

57. 656,999

58. 2,124,000

59. 456,222

60. 9,000,000

Compare the values of each of the following by inserting the greater than (>), less than (<), or equal (=) sign between the sets of whole numbers.

61. 643 ______ 762

62. 3,232 ______ 23,232

63. 654 ______ 654

64. 89,032 ______ 89,033

65. 76 ______ 67

66. 34,232 ______ 32,333

67. 323 ______ 343

68. 1 + 56 ______ 57

69. 78 – 9 ______ 69

70. 393 ______ 39 + 3

Place the following whole numbers in order beginning with the lowest value.

71. 1,234, 34,323, 54,323, 100 ____________________

72. 659, 657, 787, 343 ____________________

73. 656, 7676, 454, 654 ____________________

74. 112, 121, 211, 222 ____________________

75. 343, 342, 454, 544 ____________________

76. 343, 345, 346, 365 ____________________

77. 878, 873, 394, 493 ____________________

78. 300, 398, 382, 394 ____________________

79. 940, 483, 482, 849 ____________________

80. 984, 493, 345, 433 ____________________

Round the following numbers to the nearest ten.

81. 456 ______________________

82. 7,598 ______________________

83. 879 ______________________

84. 909 ______________________

85. 1,293 ______________________

86. 329 ______________________

87. 756 ______________________

88. 898 ______________________

89. 403 ______________________

90. 429 ______________________

Round the following numbers to the nearest hundred.

91. 3,502 ______________________

92. 54,534 ______________________

93. 34,650 ______________________

94. 1,204 ______________________

95. 78,642 ______________________

96. 23,032 ______________________

97. 4,324 ______________________

98. 55,532 ______________________

99. 98,932 ______________________

100. 430,043 ______________________

Round the following numbers to the nearest thousand.

101. 34,392 ______________________

102. 94,499 ______________________

103. 43,453 ______________________

104. 75,943 ______________________

105. 99,434 ______________________

106. 54,042 ______________________

107. 45,054 ______________________

108. 78,964 ______________________

109. 75,003 ______________________

110. 494,043 ______________________

Add the following whole numbers.

111. 12 + 2 = ______________________

112. 23 + 45 = ______________________

113. 123 + 876 = ______________________

114. 343 + 937 = ______________________

115. 67,909 + 45,433 = ______________________

116. 3,434,974 + 83,332

117. 12,232 + 513

118. 90,980 + 353,304

119. 450,032 + 393

120. 1,230,903
56,767
+ 45,322,856

Subtract the following whole numbers.

121. 456 − 76

122. 343 − 98

123. 12,576 − 989

124. 23,365 − 6,786

125. 34,327 − 6,432

126. 454,434 – 211,675 = ____________

127. 344 – 279 = ____________

128. 987 – 564 = ____________

129. 4,543 – 3,321 = ____________

130. 65,432 – 59,431 = ____________

Multiply the following whole numbers.

131. $2 \times 23 =$ ____________

132. $34 \times 231 =$ ____________

133. $432 \times 873 =$ ____________

134. $1,232 \times 430 =$ ____________

135. $1,659 \times 563 =$ ____________

136. $\begin{array}{r} 15,329 \\ \underline{\times \quad 67} \end{array}$

137. $\begin{array}{r} 35,432 \\ \underline{\times \ 9,321} \end{array}$

138. $\begin{array}{r} 459 \\ \underline{\times \ 1,321} \end{array}$

139. $\begin{array}{r} 500 \\ \underline{\times \ 124} \end{array}$

140. $\begin{array}{r} 32 \\ \underline{\times \ 783} \end{array}$

Divide the following whole numbers. Show remainders.

141. $9\overline{)45}$ ____________

142. $90\overline{)450}$ ____________

143. $80\overline{)1,239}$ ____________

144. $35\overline{)750}$ ______________________

145. $21\overline{)590}$ ______________________

146. 76,453 ÷ 293 = ______________________

147. 65,500 ÷ 25 = ______________________

148. 75,000 ÷ 360 = ______________________

149. 32 ÷ 8 = ______________________

150. 232 ÷ 4 = ______________________

Average the following whole numbers.

151. 9, 8, 9, 10, 7 ______________________

152. 12, 21, 13, 15, 20 ______________________

153. 432, 324, 456, 654, 321 ______________________

154. 90, 98, 21 ______________________

155. 900, 989, 780, 211 ______________________

156. 12,232, 24,213, 3,432, 323, 493 ______________________

157. 56, 75, 81 ______________________

158. 32, 31, 44, 34, 33, 33, 31 ______________________

159. 450, 457, 547, 543, 545 ______________________

160. 90, 99, 100, 98, 99, 96, 94, 95 ______________________

INTRODUCTION

Whether you are using Roman or Arabic numerals, it is important to understand how to add, subtract, multiply, and divide whole numbers. An understanding of these principles will help build a foundation upon which more complex operations may be performed. This chapter reviews these principles in an effort to recognize strengths and weaknesses.

Objective

4.1 Define whole number.

A **whole number** is any of the set of nonnegative integers. More clearly stated, whole numbers include zero and the counting numbers: 1, 2, 3, 4, 5, 6, 7, 8, and 9.

Objective

4.2 Explain place value of whole numbers.

Since the Arabic system of numerals utilizes ten digits (0, 1, 2, 3, 4, 5, 6, 7, 8, and 9), value is assigned by the location, or placement, of a digit within a whole number. Single digit numbers always have a place value of one. In other words, the value of the digit is the value of that digit times (multiplied by) one. When more than one digit is shown in a number, **place values** are assigned, as illustrated in Figure 4-1.

For example, if the number is 7,351, there is a 7 in the thousand's place; there is a 3 in the hundred's place; there is a 5 in the ten's place; and there is a 1 in the one's place. The number is read: seven thousand, three hundred, fifty-one.

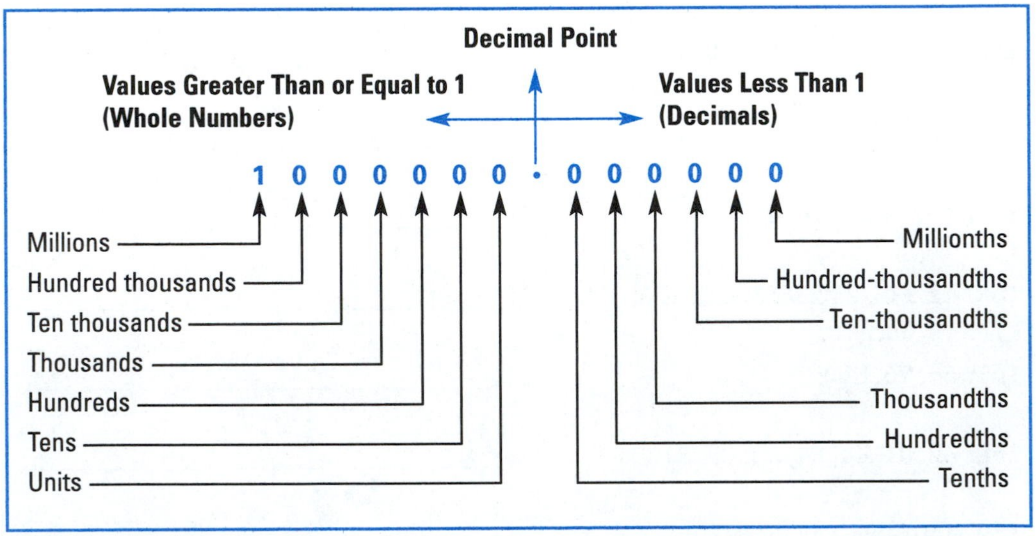

FIGURE 4-1 Place values

SKILL SHARPENER

Circle the digit in the one's place.

1. 34,506
2. 23,659
3. 123
4. 423
5. 5,463
6. 93,801
7. 912
8. 43
9. 987
10. 583

Circle the digit in the ten's place.

11. 34,506
12. 23,659
13. 123
14. 423
15. 5,463
16. 93,801
17. 912
18. 43
19. 987
20. 583

Circle the digit in the hundred's place.

21. 34,506
22. 23,659
23. 123
24. 423
25. 5,463
26. 93,801
27. 912
28. 4321
29. 987
30. 583

Circle the digit in the thousand's place.

31. 34,506
32. 23,655
33. 123,243
34. 423,970
35. 5,443
36. 93,800
37. 9,142
38. 43,899
39. 98,701
40. 500,000

Circle the digit in the ten thousand's place.

41. 34,506
42. 23,655
43. 123,900
44. 232,423
45. 55,443
46. 93,800
47. 95,212
48. 431,231
49. 987,000
50. 500,098

In each of the following problems, indicate the place value of the digit 7.

51. 234,714 ____________________

52. 745,990 ____________________

53. 234,117 ____________________

54. 111,172 ____________________

55. 1,273 ____________________

56. 795 ____________________

57. 17,980 ____________________

58. 709,932 ____________________

59. 175,000 ____________________

60. 37,500 ____________________

Objective

4.3 Compare whole numbers.

It is helpful to be able to compare the value of whole numbers. By determining whether a number is greater than, less than, or equal to another number, you can compare values of whole numbers. To compare the relative value of a whole number to another whole number, line the numbers up vertically, in rows, according to place value.

87654
86654

If one number has more digits than the other, it is the larger number. If the numbers have an equal number of digits, compare the digits starting at the left and work your way to the right, comparing each set of digits.

When you find the first set of digits that is unequal, the higher digit represents the greater number.

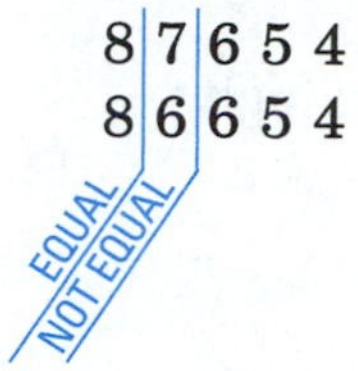

Since 7 is greater than 6, 87,654 is the larger number.

87,654 > 86,654

SKILL SHARPENER

Compare the values of each of the following by inserting the greater than (>), less than (<), or equal (=) sign between the sets of whole numbers.

1. 1,243 ______ 2,243
2. 98,211 ______ 211,098
3. 78 ______ 178
4. 987 ______ 789
5. 600,898 ______ 898,600
6. 23 ______ 24
7. 234 ______ 234
8. 372 ______ 299
9. 21,343 ______ 22,323
10. 3,320 ______ 3,430

Objective

4.4 Order whole numbers.

By comparing numbers as described in Objective 4.3, you can place numbers in order from left to right.

SKILL SHARPENER

Place the following whole numbers in order from low to high.

1. 3, 23, 54, 32, 1 ____________________

2. 67, 6, 54, 4, 16 ____________________

3. 4, 34, 35, 43, 41 ____________________

4. 7, 76, 78, 6, 5 ____________________

5. 76, 6, 54, 34, 3 ____________________

6. 9, 76, 342, 34, 21 ____________________

7. 1, 23, 456, 54, 3 ____________________

8. 2, 9, 87, 45, 3 ____________________

9. 343, 3, 43, 4, 34 ____________________

10. 342, 343, 643, 354, 454 ____________________

Objective

4.5 Round whole numbers.

When absolute precision is not required, it may be helpful to round whole numbers to the nearest ten, hundred, or thousand. For example, tongue depressors come packed in boxes of 1,000. If it is your responsibility to keep 3,000 in stock and you find that there are just over two boxes on the shelf, you would order another box of 1,000. This would be easier than counting the depressors to find that there are 2,245. By rounding 2,245 to the nearest thousand, you would find that you had approximately 2,000 depressors on the shelf and you would need to order 1,000 more.

To round whole numbers, first decide what place you will round to: the nearest ten, hundred, thousand, or so on. Once this is done, go to the place immediately to the right of the place being rounded. If this digit is 5–9, round the digit to its immediate left up one. If this digit is 0–4, leave the digit to its immediate left the same. Then change all digits to the right to zeros.

Example: Round 89 to the nearest ten.

By going to the place to the immediate right of the ten's place, we see that the digit is 9 and we should round the digit to the immediate left up one. Thus, we would round the 8 in the ten's place to a 9 and change all digits to the right to zeros, making the rounded number 90.

SKILL SHARPENER

Round each of the following numbers to the nearest ten.

1. 12 ____________________

2. 450 ____________________

3. 847 ____________________

4. 21 ____________________

5. 97 ____________________

6. 7,563 ____________________

7. 907 ____________________

8. 34 ____________________

9. 82 ____________________

10. 99 ____________________

Round each of the following numbers to the nearest hundred.

11. 1,254 ____________________

12. 989 ____________________

13. 453 ____________________

14. 265 ____________________

15. 767 ____________________

16. 9,902 ____________________

17. 457 ____________________

18. 231 ____________________

19. 109 ____________________

20. 3,982 ____________________

Round each of the following numbers to the nearest thousand.

21. 45,932 ____________________

22. 43,212 ____________________

23. 3,454 ____________________

24. 56,543 ____________________

25. 191,038 ____________________

26. 342,232 ____________________

27. 1,234 ____________________

28. 65,432 ____________________

29. 398,343 ____________________

30. 1,909 ____________________

Using the number 343,838,837,120, round to the nearest:

31. ten ____________________

32. hundred ____________________

33. thousand ____________________

34. ten thousand ____________________

35. hundred thousand ____________________

36. million ____________________

37. ten million ____________________

38. hundred million ____________________

39. billion ____________________

40. ten billion ____________________

Objective

4.6 Add whole numbers.

Addition is the process of putting numbers together. The numbers to be added are called **addends**. The answer, or total, is called the **sum**. To add whole numbers, set them up by listing the numbers to be added in a vertical format as illustrated below.

$$\begin{array}{r} 1492 \\ +\ \ 603 \\ \hline \end{array}$$

Next, add the column to the right. If the sum is 9 or lower, write the sum at the bottom of the column and move to the next column. If the sum is 10 or higher, write the last digit of the sum at the bottom of the column and carry the rest of the sum to the next column(s).

$$\begin{array}{r} 1492 \\ +\ \ 603 \\ \hline 5 \end{array}$$

2 + 3 = 5

$$\begin{array}{r} 1492 \\ +\ \ 603 \\ \hline 95 \end{array}$$

9 + 0 = 9

$$\begin{array}{r} {\scriptstyle 1} \\ 1492 \\ +\ \ 603 \\ \hline 095 \end{array}$$

4 + 6 = 10

Since the sum is 10, place 0 below the numbers being added and 1 above the next column to the left.

$$\begin{array}{r} {\scriptstyle 1} \\ 1492 \\ +\ \ 603 \\ \hline 2095 \end{array}$$

1 + 1 = 2

Continue this process until the column to the far left is added. Write the sum of this column at the bottom of the column. This reveals the sum of the equation.

SKILL SHARPENER

Find the sum.

1. 123 + 24 = ________________

2. 365 + 857 = ________________

3. 9,808 + 3,431 = ________________

4. 78 + 34 = ________________

5. 12 + 1 = ________________

6. $\begin{array}{r} 34,343 \\ +\ \ 298 \\ \hline \end{array}$

7. $\begin{array}{r} 453 \\ +\ 80 \\ \hline \end{array}$

8. $\begin{array}{r} 365 \\ +\ 2,080 \\ \hline \end{array}$

9. $\begin{array}{r} 123 \\ +\ 432 \\ \hline \end{array}$

10. $\begin{array}{r} 3,454 \\ +\ 6,755 \\ \hline \end{array}$

11. 2,398 + 34 + 196 = ________________

12. 24 + 489 + 43 = ________________

13. 243 + 87 + 1,241 = ________________

14. 212 + 32 + 100 = ________________

15. 1,265 + 3,465 + 993 + 911 = ________________

16. 2,319
564
446
+ 9,002

17. 2,003
342
+ 11

18. 32,231
3,343
4,503
+ 22,388

19. 14
62
34
+ 4,212

20. 3,342
8,766
4,459
+ 9,832

Objective

4.7 Subtract whole numbers.

Subtraction is the opposite of addition. It means to take a number away from another number. The number to be subtracted is the **subtrahend**. The number you subtract from is called the **minuend**. The answer is referred to as the **difference**.

To subtract whole numbers, set up numbers to be subtracted in vertical columns with the one's place aligned.

$$\begin{array}{r} 1632 \\ -\ 381 \\ \hline \end{array}$$

Beginning at the column on the far right, subtract the bottom digit from the top. Write the remainder below the column subtracted. If the bottom digit is larger than the top digit, you must **borrow** from the number in the next column to the left.

$$\begin{array}{r} 1632 \\ -\ 381 \\ \hline 1 \end{array}$$

$2 - 1 = 1$

In this situation, the top digit is larger than the bottom, so no borrowing is necessary. However, in the next column to the left you will have to borrow.

$$\begin{array}{r} {\scriptstyle 5\ 13} \\ 1\not{6}\not{3}2 \\ -\ \underline{381} \\ 51 \end{array}$$

13 – 8 = 5

If the digit on the bottom is larger than the digit on the top, borrow one from the digit on the top left by decreasing the digit to the left by one and adding a 1 (representing 10) to the left of the digit in question. Rather than attempting to subtract 3 – 8, now subtract 13 – 8. Place your answer in the space below the equation.

$$\begin{array}{r} {\scriptstyle 5\ 13} \\ 1\not{6}\not{3}2 \\ -\ \underline{381} \\ 251 \end{array}$$

5 – 3 = 2

Continue subtracting by moving to the left.

$$\begin{array}{r} {\scriptstyle 5\ 13} \\ 1\not{6}\not{3}2 \\ -\ \underline{381} \\ 1251 \end{array}$$

1 – 0 = 1

SKILL SHARPENER

Find the difference.

1. 12 – 3

2. 143 – 25

3. 1,298 – 345

4. 184,403 – 2,678

5. 989,987 – 232,432

6. 74,532 – 34,002

7. 989 – 31 = ______________

8. 435 – 98 = ______________

9. 7,342,343 – 56,433 = ______________

10. 90,980 – 21,232 = ______________

Objective

4.8 Multiply whole numbers.

Multiplication allows you to quickly add like numbers. For example, rather than adding the following column of numbers, it is easier to multiply.

$$\begin{array}{r} 6 \\ 6 \\ 6 \\ 6 \\ 6 \\ +\ 6 \\ \hline 36 \end{array}$$

OR $6 \times 6 = 36$

The numbers being multiplied are called **factors**. The specific terms, **multiplicand** and **multiplier**, are sometimes used to differentiate the number being multiplied and the number the multiplicand is being multiplied by. The result is known as the **product**.

To multiply whole numbers, set up numbers to be multiplied in vertical columns with the one's place aligned.

$$\begin{array}{r} 131 \\ \times\ 18 \\ \hline \end{array}$$

Begin by multiplying the digits in the far right column. If the product is 9 or less, write the product in the space below that column. If the product is 10 or higher, write the last digit of the product in the space below the column and write the first digit above the top number in the next column to the left.

$$\begin{array}{r} 131 \\ \times\ 18 \\ \hline 8 \end{array}$$

$1 \times 8 = 8$

While continuing to use the number to the right of the bottom number, multiply it by the number in the next column to the left, on the top. Then add any remaining amount that you may have noted above the top number. Continue with these steps until you have multiplied each column by the digit in the one's place.

$$\begin{array}{r} {}^{2}\ \ \ \\ 131 \\ \times\ 18 \\ \hline 48 \end{array}$$

$3 \times 8 = 24$

$$\begin{array}{r} {}^{2}\ \ \ \\ 131 \\ \times\ 18 \\ \hline 1048 \end{array}$$

$1 \times 8 = 8 + 2 = 10$

Now repeat the process for the digit in the tens place, aligning your answer beginning with the tens place on a row beneath the first row of answers.

$$\begin{array}{r} 131 \\ \times\ 18 \\ \hline 1048 \\ 1 \end{array}$$

$1 \times 1 = 1$

$$\begin{array}{r} 131 \\ \times\ 18 \\ \hline 1048 \\ 31 \end{array}$$

$3 \times 1 = 3$

$$\begin{array}{r} 131 \\ \times\ 18 \\ \hline 1048 \\ 131 \end{array}$$

$1 \times 1 = 1$

Once all the multiplication has been done, add the answers to reveal the product.

$$\begin{array}{r} 131 \\ \times\ 18 \\ \hline 1048 \\ +\ 131 \\ \hline 2358 \end{array}$$

SKILL SHARPENER

Find the product.

1. 12 × 34 = ____________________

2. 253 × 654 = ____________________

3. 345 × 298 = ____________________

4. 732,343 × 392 = ____________________

5. $\begin{array}{r} 25{,}767 \\ \times\ 900{,}012 \\ \hline \end{array}$

6. $\begin{array}{r} 1{,}203 \\ \times\ 89 \\ \hline \end{array}$

7. $\begin{array}{r} 450 \\ \times\ 392 \\ \hline \end{array}$

8. 232,343
× 898,483

9. 5,654,788
× 7

10. 45,009
× 34

Objective

4.9 Divide whole numbers.

Division is the opposite of multiplication. That is, it is the process of determining how many times one number is found within another number. The number being divided is called the **dividend.** The number divided into the dividend is called the **divisor**. The answer is referred to as the **quotient**. If there is part of the dividend that is not divided, it is called the **remainder**.

Let's try an example to illustrate that division is the opposite of multiplication. We know that 6 × 3 = 18. Now we will set this up as we would set up a division problem.

$$6\overline{)18}\quad \text{quotient } 3$$

6 × 3 = 18
3 × 6 = 18

We also know, from looking at this example, that 18 ÷ 6 = 3 and 18 ÷ 3 = 6. But what happens when one of the factors is removed?

By removing the known factor of 3, we now have a division problem illustrated as:

18 ÷ 6 = _____

This is set up as:

$$6\overline{)18}$$

Since we know that our missing factor is 3, we can easily solve this problem.

$$6\overline{)18}\quad \text{quotient } 3$$

But what if the missing factor is not so obvious? In this case, begin by estimating the quotient.

25 ÷ 4 = _____

Set up as:

$$4\overline{)25}$$

Now estimate the dividend. Since we know that 6 × 4 = 24, we can determine that the dividend will be approximately 6. Therefore, place a 6 over the 25.

$$\begin{array}{r} 6 \\ 4\overline{)25} \end{array}$$

Now multiply 6 × 4.
The answer is 24. Place a 24 under the 25.

$$\begin{array}{r} 6 \\ 4\overline{)25} \\ 24 \end{array}$$

Now subtract 25 – 24.
The answer is 1.

$$\begin{array}{r} 6 \\ 4\overline{)25} \\ \underline{24} \\ 1 \end{array}$$

Therefore, the answer to the problem 25 ÷ 6 = __ is 4 with a remainder of 1.

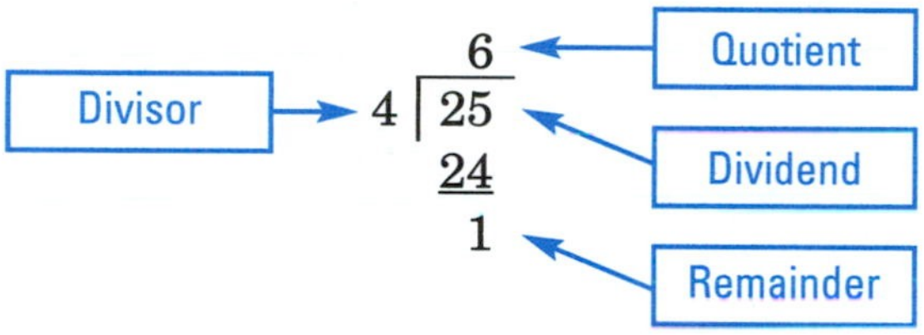

What if the problem is larger, like 129 ÷ 5?

The problem:

129 ÷ 5 = _____

Set up as:

$$5\overline{)129}$$

Estimate. We can begin by estimating that 5 will go into 12 two times. Since you are dividing into 12, place the 2 over the 12.

$$\begin{array}{r} 2 \\ 5\overline{)129} \end{array}$$

Now multiply 5 × 2 = 10.

$$\begin{array}{r} 2 \\ 5\overline{)129} \\ 10 \end{array}$$

Subtract 12 – 10 = 2.

$$\begin{array}{r} 2 \\ 5\overline{)129} \\ -\underline{10} \\ 2 \end{array}$$

Bring down the 9.

$$\begin{array}{r} 2 \\ 5\overline{)129} \\ \underline{10}\downarrow \\ 29 \end{array}$$

Now divide 5 into 29.

$$\begin{array}{r} 2 \\ 5\overline{)129} \\ \underline{10} \\ 29 \end{array}$$

Since we know that 5 × 5 = 25, we will use 5.

$$\begin{array}{r} 25 \\ 5\overline{)129} \\ \underline{10} \\ 29 \\ \underline{25} \end{array}$$

Subtract 29 – 25 = 4.

$$\begin{array}{r} 25 \\ 5\overline{)129} \\ \underline{10} \\ 29 \\ -\underline{25} \\ 4 \end{array}$$

Solution: 129 ÷ 5 = 25 with a remainder of 4.

Check your answer by multiplying the quotient by the divisor. Your answer should be the same as the dividend. When a remainder is present, multiply the quotient by the divisor, then add the remainder.

$$\begin{array}{r} 5 \times 25 = 125 \\ \underline{+\ \ 4} \\ 129 \end{array}$$

← Remainder

SKILL SHARPENER

Find the quotient. Show remainders.

1. 24 ÷ 4 = ____________________

2. 7,393 ÷ 345 = ____________________

3. 783,343 ÷ 938 = ____________________

4. 75,000 ÷ 25 = ____________________

5. 78,932 ÷ 431 = ____________________

6. $900\overline{)394{,}322{,}300}$ ____________________

7. $5\overline{)650}$ ____________________

8. $60\overline{)125{,}000}$ ____________________

9. $234\overline{)57{,}876}$ ____________________

10. $12\overline{)975{,}034{,}302}$ ____________________

Objective

4.10 Average whole numbers.

An **average** is a mathematical **mean**. To average whole numbers, find the sum of all of the numbers in the set and divide by the number that makes up the set.

The problem: Average the following set of numbers:

94, 87, 98, 79

Add.

$$\begin{array}{r} 94 \\ 87 \\ 98 \\ +\ 79 \\ \hline 358 \end{array}$$

Divide by the number in the set.

$358 \div 4 = 89.5$

Solution: Mathematic average, or mean, is 89.5.

SKILL SHARPENER

Average the following sets of whole numbers.

1. 90, 92, 98, 100, 100, 78 ____________

2. 87, 43, 345, 43, 34, 344 ____________

3. 120, 220, 323, 323, 210 ____________

4. 321, 983, 343, 3,433, 322 ____________

5. 909, 900, 908, 906, 911 ____________

6. 75, 65, 34, 94, 32, 234 ____________

7. 12,332, 23,322, 3,443 ____________

8. 334, 3,464, 4,603 ____________

9. 8,575, 4,933, 939 ____________

10. 39,393, 932, 3,985 ____________

CONCLUSION

As a health care provider, part of your daily routine will involve applying the mathematical skills you have learned. Whether you are measuring intake and output or performing drug calculations, your ability to perform basic computations using whole numbers is important and will help you to perform more complicated computations.

REVIEW AND REFLECT

1. What is a whole number?

2. Why is it important to understand the place values of whole numbers?

3. Give an example of when whole numbers might need to be rounded.

4. Why is it helpful to be able to average whole numbers?

5. What is another word for average?

CHAPTER 5

Decimals

LEARNING OBJECTIVES

After completing this chapter, the reader will be able to:

- **5.1** Define decimals.
- **5.2** Explain place value of decimals.
- **5.3** Explain advantages of using decimals.
- **5.4** Compare decimals.
- **5.5** Round decimals.
- **5.6** Add decimals.
- **5.7** Subtract decimals.
- **5.8** Multiply decimals.
- **5.9** Divide decimals.
- **5.10** Average decimals.

KEY TERM

- decimal

MATH IN THE REAL WORLD

"If I am to give an injection of 50 mg of Demerol but only have 100 mg/mL doses available, I would use decimals to learn I need to administer 0.5 mL."

Joyce Mitchell, RN

SELF-ASSESSMENT **PRETEST**

Circle the digit found in the one's place.

1. 45.34

2. 690.00

3. 212.932

4. 32.893

5. 785.112

6. 3,215.190

7. 9,950.250

8. 451.364

9. 34,590.773

10. 23,321.500

Circle the digit found in the tenth's place.

11. 54.980

12. 6,790.3532

13. 356.121

14. 100.56

15. 4,341.5550

16. 67,650.341

17. 900.9000

18. 15,250.375

19. 8.375

20. 100.875

Circle the digit found in the hundredth's place.

21. 34.1230

22. 500.3209

23. 65.9010

24. 750.8793

25. 3,500.5300

26. 353.1250

27. 795.975

28. 900.01991

29. 63,475.9801

30. 7,601.9000

Circle the digit in the thousandth's place.

31. 540.3421

32. 442.3928

33. 7,988.8897

34. 452.5203

35. 32,321.902

36. 431.23179

37. 299.2020

38. 29.20232

39. 365.245

40. 943.7075

Compare the following numbers by placing the greater than ($>$), less than ($<$), or equal to ($=$) sign in the blank.

41. 325.99 _____ 392.343

42. 25.11 _____ 25.1100

43. 65.120 _____ 65.12

44. 900.01 _____ 901.100

45. 645.321 _____ 645.0321

46. 7.9500 _____ 7.905

47. 81.245 _____ 81.0245

48. 9.012 _____ 9.0120

49. 34.321 _____ 34.3211

50. 90.09 _____ 90.090

Round the following numbers to the nearest tenth.

51. 34.3254 ____________

52. 12.393 ____________

53. 453.9044 ____________

54. 45.433 ____________

55. 475.755 ____________

56. 939.30 ____________

57. 948.4 ____________

58. 397.33 ____________

59. 94,847.884 ____________

60. 948.47 ____________

Round the following numbers to the nearest hundredth.

61. 8,347.474 ____________

62. 34.32221 ____________

63. 455.4454 ____________

64. 499.9595 ____________

65. 595.5943 ____________

66. 4.454 ____________

67. 45.4387 ____________

68. 995.553 ____________

69. 454.441 ____________

70. 9,045.443 ____________

Round the following numbers to the nearest thousandth.

71. 3,433.33434 ____________

72. 44.40404 ____________

73. 434.4443 ____________

74. 8.6452 ____________

75. 0.3331 ____________

76. 102.2332 ____________

77. 3.3433 ____________

78. 6.4543 ____________

79. 4.5401 ____________

80. 9.4045 ____________

Add the following.

81. 34.32 + 343.23 = ______________

82. 454.32 + 32.01 = ______________

83. 904.432 + 323.333 = ______________

84. 9.343 + 45.433 = ______________

85. 354,334.3984 + 12.3 = ______________

86. 493.3 + 948.43 = ______________

87. 454.433
+ 9,448.4

88. 98,433.001
+ 1,232.39409

89. 765.434
+ 43.200

90. 938.40
+ 34

Subtract the following.

91. 34.532
− 0.543

92. 5.440
− 2.333

93. 975.431
− 543.94943

94. 90.43
− 89.49

95. 454.342 − 398.329 = ____________________

96. 9,484.12 − 56.2 = ____________________

97. 875.320 − 865.321 = ____________________

98. 1.25 − 0.94 = ____________________

99. 5,943.4034 − 34.432 = ____________________

100. 47.43 − 45.44 = ____________________

Multiply the following.

101. 747.12 × 94 = ____________________

102. 9.03 × 12.2 = ____________________

103. 453,439.9334 × 393.49332 = ____________________

104. 4,543.3444 × 93,030.9302 = ____________________

105. 373.39383
× 990.3

106. 12.23
× 6

107. 8,474.493
× 837

108. 94,873
$\times$ 9.42

109. 737
$\times$ 9.03

110. 34.32
$\times$ 93

Divide the following.

111. 12 ÷ 3.22 = __________

112. 493 ÷ 323.32 = __________

113. 121.200 ÷ 89 = __________

114. 334.332 ÷ 39.30 = __________

115. 398.39 ÷ 32.1 = __________

116. $303.3\overline{)759.32}$

117. $39.32\overline{)750.21}$

118. $28.23\overline{)32}$

119. $34.321\overline{)833.43}$

120. $834.3\overline{)3{,}939.33}$

Average the following sets of numbers.

121. 23.323, 34.3, 454.432, 984.422, 94.43 ______________________

122. 83.32, 304.03, 12.51, 34.343, 329.43 ______________________

123. 90.322, 91.323, 89.998, 93.23 ______________________

124. 765.42, 764.66, 464.44, 65.422 ______________________

125. 911.21, 900.21, 901.22, 890.322, 900.21 ______________________

126. 12.212, 321.232, 232.22, 42.32, 23.222 ______________________

127. 9.99, 9.978, 9.987, 9.901, 9.021 ______________________

128. 4.454, 4.54, 4.4, 4.561, 4.544 ______________________

129. 2.323, 2.343, 3.332, 323.33 ______________________

130. 5.43, 4.3432, 3.4464, 6.453, 3.9935 ______________________

INTRODUCTION

Health care providers utilize decimals on a daily basis for anything from preparing medications to paying for lunch. Knowledge of the decimal system will help you to perform a variety of everyday tasks.

Objective

5.1 Define decimals.

A **decimal** represents a fraction of a whole number whose denominators are multiples of 10. For example, 0.65 represents 65 hundredths and could be represented as 65/100.

Objective

5.2 Explain place value of decimals.

Like whole numbers, decimals have place values. Since the digits to the left of the decimal are whole numbers, the place values are ones, tens, hundreds, thousands, and so on. The place values to the right of the decimal represent portions of one and include tenth, hundredth, thousandth, and so on as represented in Figure 5-1.

For example, the number 145.679 represents the whole number one hundred forty-five and 679 thousandths. One of the most common uses of decimals is in our monetary system where we deal with dollars and cents. Nine hundred sixty-three dollars and thirty-seven cents is represented as $963.37. Another way to say this amount is nine hundred sixty-three and thirty-seven hundredths. Using decimals makes it easier to recognize, add, subtract, multiply, and divide numbers with fractional amounts.

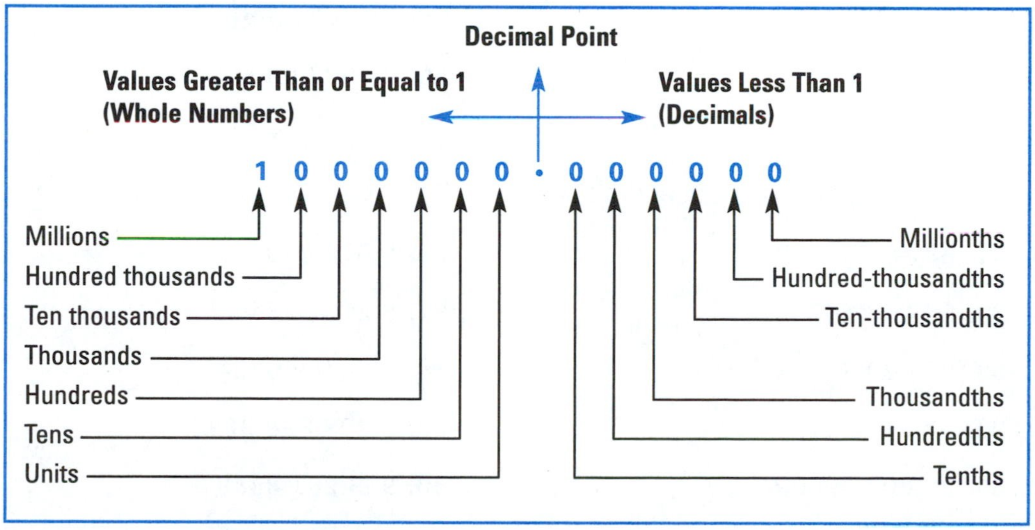

FIGURE 5-1 Comparing decimals

SKILL SHARPENER

Circle the digit in the one's place.

1. 123.00
2. 98.37
3. 21.938
4. 39.09
5. 2,222.222
6. 78.90
7. 34.67
8. 87.67
9. 12.789
10. 865.432

Circle the digit in the tenth's place.

11. 56.9987
12. 884.09
13. 9,292.77382
14. 478,333.929
15. 993.909
16. 848.9309
17. 758.423
18. 7,583,902.0752
19. 9,832.9853
20. 10,000,007.3

Circle the digit in the hundredth's place

21. 8,437.0303
22. 12,267.009772
23. 487.0932
24. 9.341876
25. 4,576.888
26. 32,907,458.1208743
27. 8,594.90329
28. 48.444
29. 982.030908
30. 90,003.00000007

Circle the digit in the thousandth's place

31. 637,367.8969
32. 988,989.434233
33. 895.2090
34. 57,847.0549
35. 20,009.00009
36. 8,578.489
37. 8,578.9834
38. 598,489.93843
39. 3,298,398.9696
40. 989,201.3489765

Objective

5.3 Explain advantages of using decimals.

Since the decimal system is divisible by ten, it allows for easy recognition, comparison, and calculation of very large numbers. Since our monetary system utilizes the decimal system, most of us are familiar with common mathematical applications used in making purchases, writing checks, paying bills, and balancing our checkbooks.

SKILL SHARPENER

Write the following numbers using decimals. Then decide which is easier to read and understand: the way you wrote them or the way they are written here.

Decimals

1. One hundred seventy-five and ninety-eight hundredths ____________
2. Seven thousand forty-three and seven hundred forty-two thousandths ____________
3. Ninety-nine thousand three hundred forty-nine and sixty-seven hundredths ____________
4. Thirty-three and ninety hundredths ____________
5. Seventeen and seven thousand six hundred thirty-one ten-thousandths ____________
6. Ninety-nine dollars and fifty-nine cents ____________
7. Three thousand nine hundred forty-three dollars and thirty-two cents ____________
8. Forty-five dollars and sixteen cents ____________
9. Three thousand sixty dollars and fifty-three cents ____________
10. Nine hundred ninety-three dollars and four cents ____________

Objective

5.4 Compare decimals.

Decimals are compared by observing the digits in each place, beginning at the far left. Continue to the right until you find digits that are unequal. At that point, the larger digit represents the the larger number.

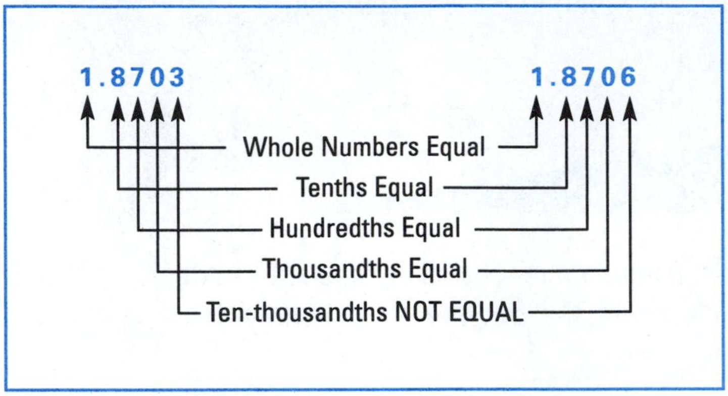

SKILL SHARPENER

Compare the following decimals by placing the greater than (>), less than (<), or equal to (=) sign in the blank.

1. 0000003.000003 _______ 0000003.0000003

2. 187.567 _______ 187.68

3. 65.76 _______ 64.78

4. 4,753.8473 _______ 4,753.74938

5. 7,483.1 _______ 7,483.99999

6. 9,485.09383 _______ 9,485.09384

7. 2,399.8940 _______ 2,399.894

8. 748.737 _______ 748.747

9. .5000000 _______ .5

10. 878.870 _______ 878.8700000

Objective

5.5 Round decimals.

Decimal numbers may be rounded in the same way that whole numbers are rounded. First, determine what place you will round to: the nearest tenth, hundredth, thousandth, or so on. Look one place to the right of the place being rounded. If this digit is 5–9, round the digit to its immediate left up one and drop all the digits to the right of the place you are rounding. If the digit is 0–4, leave the digit to its immediate left the same and drop all digits to the right of the place you are rounding.

Example: Round 345.9672 to the nearest hundredth.

The 6 is in the hundredth's place. Since there is a 7 to the right of the hundredth's place, round the hundredth's place up to 7 and drop all digits to the right of the hundredth's place. Your answer is 345.97.

Example: Round 45.27314 to the nearest thousandth.

If your answer is 45.273, you are correct. Since the digit to the right of the thousandth's place is less than 5, leave the thousandth's place the same and drop the digits to the right.

SKILL SHARPENER

Round to the nearest tenth.

1. 843.839 ______________

2. 7,483.09 ______________

3. 728.89 ______________

4. 97.09 ______________

5. 13.435 ______________

6. 8,392.9209 ______________

7. 574,837.384982 ______________

8. 83.3989 ______________

9. 84,398.839 ______________

10. 9,389.849 ______________

Round to the nearest hundredth.

11. 8,437.48394 ____________________

12. 38,378.89384 ____________________

13. 22.2222 ____________________

14. 43.432 ____________________

15. 4,903.695 ____________________

16. 829.8509 ____________________

17. 9,303.3093 ____________________

18. 15,940.9303 ____________________

19. 302.940 ____________________

20. 1,515.425 ____________________

Round to the nearest thousandth.

21. 78.93899 ____________________

22. 5,874.9806 ____________________

23. 93,939.065555 ____________________

24. 8,097.324132 ____________________

25. 8,439.5241 ____________________

26. 987,432.7094 ____________________

27. 098.4325222222 ____________________

28. 90,776,890.345209 ____________________

29. 998,432,497.5848 ____________________

30. 2.66666 ____________________

Objective

5.6 Add decimals.

Decimals are added like whole numbers. To set up the problem, line up the decimals and add normally. Bring the decimal straight down.

The problem:

72.8 + 3.1 = ______

Set up as:

```
  72.8
+  3.1
```

Add as you would whole numbers.

```
  72.8
+  3.1
  75.9
```

Solution: 72.8 + 3.1 = 75.9

SKILL SHARPENER

Add the following decimals.

1. 4.5 + 8.4 = ______________________

2. 3.2 + 8.6 = ______________________

3. 89.22 + 77.56 = ______________________

4. 584.9 + 784.99 = ______________________

5. 232.64 + 346.98 = ______________________

6.
```
  674.854
+  84.874
```

7.
```
  6.7
  8.9
  2.8
  9.0
+ 4.5
```

8.
```
   747.748
   848.398
+ 8,327.82
```

9. 777.9
878.8
+ 7,832.378

10. 2.3
5.6
+ 7.9

Objective

5.7 Subtract decimals.

Set up the problem with decimals aligned. Subtract as you would a whole number, borrowing when necessary. Bring the decimal straight down to reveal the answer.

The problem:

$$48.2 - 7.1 = \_\_\_\_\_$$

Set up as:

$$\begin{array}{r} 48.2 \\ -\quad 7.1 \\ \hline \end{array}$$

Subtract as you would whole numbers.

$$\begin{array}{r} 48.2 \\ -\quad 7.1 \\ \hline 41.1 \end{array}$$

Solution: 48.2 − 7.1 = 41.1

SKILL SHARPENER

Subtract the following decimals.

1. 5.6
− 3.2

2. 8,774.885
− 784.44

3. $\begin{array}{r} 8{,}889.33 \\ -\ 4{,}332.43 \\ \hline \end{array}$

4. $\begin{array}{r} 14.5 \\ -\ 5.2 \\ \hline \end{array}$

5. $\begin{array}{r} 100{,}982.292 \\ -\ 94{,}398.99 \\ \hline \end{array}$

6. $\begin{array}{r} 889.94 \\ -\ 757.88 \\ \hline \end{array}$

7. 5,894.94 − 4,783.84 = ______________________

8. 849.849 − 58.84 = ______________________

9. 954.9 − 944.98 = ______________________

10. 8,754.94 − 88.8 = ______________________

Objective

5.8 Multiply decimals.

Set up your problems as you would whole numbers. Decimals do not need to be aligned. Multiply normally. Count the combined number of decimal places in the factors and move the decimal in your product from right to left that number of places.

The problem:

$$12.8 \times 1.3 = \underline{\qquad}$$

Set up as:

$$\begin{array}{r} 12.8 \\ \times\ 1.3 \\ \hline \end{array}$$

Multiply as you would whole numbers.

$$\begin{array}{r} 12.8 \\ \times\ 1.3 \\ \hline 384 \\ 128 \\ \hline 1664 \end{array}$$

Move decimal to the left the total number of places in the factors.

```
  12.8   ← One place
×  1.3   ← One place
  384
 128
 16.64   ← Move two places
```

Solution: 12.8 × 1.3 = 16.64

SKILL SHARPENER

Multiply the following decimals.

1. 89.54 × 849.84 = ______________________

2. 8,493.4839 × 884.489 = ______________________

3. 933.84 × 944.3789 = ______________________

4. 448.84 × 8,493.389 = ______________________

5. 9,389.84 × 493.847

6. 893.2283 × 89.493

7. 490.09 × 84.84

8. 3.4 × 44.7

9. 9,039.49 × 748.8

10. 895,849.9595 × 7,584.89389

Objective

5.9 Divide decimals.

To divide decimals, set up your problem as shown here.

The problem:

$$59.15 \div 6.5 = \_\_\_\_\_\_$$

Set up equation as:

$$6.5\overline{)59.15}$$

Move decimal in the divisor to the right to make the divisor a whole number. Then move the decimal in the dividend to the right the same number of places.

Place decimal on answer line.

$$6.5\overline{)59.15}$$

Divide as you would whole numbers.

```
       9.1
65 ) 591.5
     585
       65
       65
       00
```

Solution: 59.15 ÷ 6.5 = 9.1

SKILL SHARPENER

Divide the following decimals.

1. 8,877.9 ÷ 6.25 = ________________

2. 4,355.5 ÷ 12.5 = ________________

3. 15.35 ÷ 0.5 = ________________

4. 848.59 ÷ 100.2 = ________________

5. $12.1\overline{)36.48}$ ________________

6. $6.25\overline{)98.1}$ ________________

7. $8.94\overline{)89.4}$ ________________

8. $4\overline{)38.65}$ ______________________

9. $5\overline{)485.625}$ ______________________

10. $3\overline{)90.54}$ ______________________

Objective

5.10 Average decimals.

To average decimals, first find the sum of the numbers in the set. Then, divide that sum by the quantity of numbers in the set. This is your average.

The problem:

Average the following set of numbers: 90.3, 92.1, 91.3, 94.8.

Set up equation as:

$$\begin{array}{r} 90.3 \\ 92.1 \\ 91.3 \\ +\ 94.8 \\ \hline \end{array}$$

Find the sum.

$$\begin{array}{r} \overset{1}{9}0.3 \\ 92.1 \\ 91.3 \\ +\ \ 94.8 \\ \hline 368.5 \end{array}$$

Divide the sum by the quantity of numbers in the set.

$$\begin{array}{r|l} & 92.125 \\ \hline 4 & 368.5 \\ & \underline{36} \\ & 08 \\ & \underline{\ 8} \\ & \quad 5 \\ & \quad \underline{4} \\ & \quad 10 \\ & \quad \ \underline{8} \\ & \quad \ 20 \\ & \quad \ \underline{20} \\ & \quad \ \ 0 \end{array}$$

Solution: 92.125

SKILL SHARPENER

Average the following numbers.

1. 6.7, 6.8, 6.4, 5.9 ____________________

2. 344.4, 345.2, 341.5, 339.8 ____________________

3. 1.1, 2.7, 4.7, 8.5, 3.6 ____________________

4. 4,555.554, 4,557.552, 4,549.553 ____________________

5. 18.9, 20.3, 17.5, 21.7, 17.3 ____________________

6. 90.3, 100, 99.9, 94.4, 96.7, 98.3 ____________________

7. 55.5, 53.6, 52.9, 56.7 ____________________

8. 6.5, 10.8, 5.3, 7.9, 9.9 ____________________

9. 7.8, 9.0, 8.4, 5.3, 7.4 ____________________

10. 433.66, 434.5, 430.8, 436.8 ____________________

CONCLUSION

Decimals are part of everyday life. Whether you are paying bills, buying lunch, mixing or administering medications, or reviewing your paycheck for accuracy, you will utilize your knowledge of the decimal system. This knowledge and the skills you have learned in this chapter will help you to function better, not only in your job, but also in everyday life.

REVIEW AND REFLECT

1. Discuss ways to use decimals in everyday life.

____

____

____

____

____

2. Discuss the advantages of using decimals.

3. How can you easily multiply a decimal by 10, 100, 1,000, and so on?

4. How can you easily divide a decimal by 10, 100, 1,000, and so on?

5. Why are the operations described in questions 3 and 4 possible?

CHAPTER

6

Fractions

LEARNING OBJECTIVES

After completing this chapter, the reader will be able to:

- 6.1 Define fractions.
- 6.2 Explain advantages of using fractions.
- 6.3 Find the numerator.
- 6.4 Find the denominator.
- 6.5 Order fractions.
- 6.6 Add fractions with common denominators.
- 6.7 Subtract fractions with common denominators.
- 6.8 Define mixed number.
- 6.9 Add mixed numbers with common denominators.
- 6.10 Subtract mixed numbers with common denominators.
- 6.11 Define factors.
- 6.12 Find common factors.
- 6.13 Find the greatest common factor.
- 6.14 Reduce fractions.
- 6.15 Define proper fraction.
- 6.16 Define improper fraction.
- 6.17 Change improper fractions to proper fractions.
- 6.18 Define multiple.
- 6.19 Define least common multiple.

KEY TERMS

- canceling
- common denominator
- common factor
- denominator
- factor
- fraction
- greatest common factor (GCF)
- improper fraction
- least common denominator (LCD)
- least common multiple (LCM)
- mixed number
- multiple
- numerator
- proper fraction
- uncommon denominator
- uncommon factor

- **6.20** Find the least common denominator.
- **6.21** Add fractions with uncommon denominators.
- **6.22** Subtract fractions with uncommon denominators.
- **6.23** Use borrowing to subtract fractions.
- **6.24** Change mixed numbers to improper fractions.
- **6.25** Multiply fractions.
- **6.26** Multiply fractions using canceling.
- **6.27** Multiply fractions and whole numbers.
- **6.28** Multiply fractions and mixed numbers.
- **6.29** Divide fractions.

MATH IN THE REAL WORLD

"We use fractions for exposure factors...as by increasing or decreasing an exposure..."

Barbara Hammond, Radiology Assistant

SELF-ASSESSMENT **PRETEST**

Circle the numerator in the following fractions.

1. $\frac{1}{2}$
2. $\frac{23}{48}$
3. $\frac{2}{10}$
4. $\frac{6}{12}$
5. $\frac{125}{1,000}$
6. $\frac{15}{90}$
7. $\frac{2}{900}$
8. $\frac{45}{500}$
9. $\frac{6}{9}$
10. $\frac{180}{360}$

Circle the denominator in the following fractions.

11. $\frac{12}{14}$
12. $\frac{5}{61}$
13. $\frac{15}{16}$
14. $\frac{7}{8}$
15. $\frac{3}{4}$
16. $\frac{325}{650}$
17. $\frac{9}{12}$
18. $\frac{500}{15,000}$
19. $\frac{4}{16}$
20. $\frac{17}{18}$

Place the following fractions in order from smallest to largest.

21. $\frac{1}{2}$ $\frac{1}{3}$ $\frac{1}{4}$ $\frac{1}{5}$ $\frac{1}{6}$ ____________________
22. $\frac{7}{16}$ $\frac{3}{8}$ $\frac{1}{2}$ $\frac{9}{16}$ $\frac{3}{4}$ ____________________
23. $\frac{12}{15}$ $\frac{12}{16}$ $\frac{9}{10}$ $\frac{11}{16}$ $\frac{7}{8}$ ____________________
24. $\frac{6}{15}$ $\frac{4}{9}$ $\frac{10}{12}$ $\frac{3}{4}$ $\frac{4}{5}$ ____________________
25. $\frac{1}{2}$ $\frac{2}{3}$ $\frac{3}{4}$ $\frac{4}{5}$ $\frac{5}{6}$ ____________________
26. $\frac{5}{8}$ $\frac{6}{8}$ $\frac{3}{16}$ $\frac{9}{32}$ $\frac{7}{64}$ ____________________
27. $\frac{15}{16}$ $\frac{13}{16}$ $\frac{7}{8}$ $\frac{9}{14}$ $\frac{2}{3}$ ____________________
28. $\frac{4}{7}$ $\frac{9}{15}$ $\frac{2}{45}$ $\frac{5}{75}$ $\frac{4}{5}$ ____________________
29. $\frac{7}{8}$ $\frac{12}{15}$ $\frac{9}{16}$ $\frac{13}{16}$ $\frac{2}{3}$ ____________________
30. $\frac{17}{24}$ $\frac{3}{8}$ $\frac{8}{12}$ $\frac{4}{5}$ $\frac{8}{100}$ ____________________

Add the following fractions with common denominators.

31. $\frac{1}{3} + \frac{2}{3} =$ __________

32. $\frac{3}{4} + \frac{1}{4} =$ __________

33. $\frac{15}{16} + \frac{2}{16} =$ __________

34. $\frac{3}{12} + \frac{2}{12} =$ __________

35. $\frac{6}{64} + \frac{12}{64} =$ __________

36. $\frac{1}{5} + \frac{3}{5} =$ __________

37. $\frac{1}{100} + \frac{54}{100} =$ __________

38. $\frac{45}{50} + \frac{3}{50} =$ __________

39. $\frac{15}{60} + \frac{30}{60} =$ __________

40. $\frac{9}{144} + \frac{3}{144} =$ __________

Subtract the following fractions with common denominators.

41. $\frac{12}{100} - \frac{10}{100} =$ __________

42. $\frac{98}{144} - \frac{62}{144} =$ __________

43. $\frac{9}{10} - \frac{6}{10} =$ __________

44. $\frac{3}{4} - \frac{1}{4} =$ __________

45. $\frac{4}{5} - \frac{2}{5} =$ __________

46. $\frac{12}{16} - \frac{4}{16} =$ __________

47. $\frac{45}{50} - \frac{40}{50} =$ __________

48. $\frac{34}{36} - \frac{4}{36} =$ ______________

49. $\frac{150}{600} - \frac{7}{600} =$ ______________

50. $\frac{35}{75} - \frac{5}{75} =$ ______________

Add the following mixed numbers with common denominators.

51. $1\frac{2}{3} + 2\frac{1}{3} =$ ______________

52. $1\frac{15}{16} + 2\frac{3}{16} =$ ______________

53. $23\frac{1}{2} + 4\frac{1}{2} =$ ______________

54. $12\frac{4}{5} + 6\frac{1}{5} =$ ______________

55. $2\frac{1}{8} + 3\frac{3}{8} =$ ______________

56. $3\frac{6}{10} + 2\frac{9}{10} =$ ______________

57. $51\frac{4}{8} + 2\frac{2}{8} =$ ______________

58. $9\frac{1}{9} + 1\frac{1}{9} =$ ______________

59. $4\frac{6}{9} + 1\frac{1}{9} =$ ______________

60. $34\frac{1}{90} + 2\frac{76}{90} =$ ______________

Subtract the following mixed numbers with common denominators.

61. $23\frac{1}{4} - 12\frac{3}{4} =$ ______________

62. $56\frac{1}{4} - 2\frac{3}{4} =$ ______________

63. $1\frac{15}{16} - 1\frac{2}{16} =$ ______________

64. $39\frac{7}{8} - 3\frac{2}{8} =$ ______________

65. $13\frac{2}{5} - 2\frac{3}{5} =$ ______________________

66. $6\frac{9}{100} - 2\frac{34}{100} =$ ______________________

67. $33\frac{1}{3} - 3\frac{2}{3} =$ ______________________

68. $6\frac{45}{50} - 3\frac{2}{50} =$ ______________________

69. $7\frac{2}{7} - 2\frac{5}{7} =$ ______________________

70. $8\frac{2}{8} - 3\frac{5}{8} =$ ______________________

Find the factors for the following numbers.

71. 12 ______________________

72. 16 ______________________

73. 6 ______________________

74. 10 ______________________

75. 8 ______________________

76. 14 ______________________

77. 32 ______________________

78. 7 ______________________

79. 4 ______________________

80. 18 ______________________

Find the greatest common factor of the following pairs of numbers.

81. 12, 18 ______________________

82. 6, 12 ______________________

83. 9, 12 ______________________

84. 8, 16 ______________________

85. 12, 16 ______________________

86. 32, 14 ______________________

87. 12, 32 ______________________

88. 9, 18 ______________________

89. 4, 20 ______________________

90. 24, 36 ______________________

Reduce the following fractions.

91. $\frac{9}{18}$ ____________

92. $\frac{8}{24}$ ____________

93. $\frac{2}{32}$ ____________

94. $\frac{15}{45}$ ____________

95. $\frac{21}{24}$ ____________

96. $\frac{20}{32}$ ____________

97. $\frac{45}{50}$ ____________

98. $\frac{80}{100}$ ____________

99. $\frac{2}{6}$ ____________

100. $\frac{6}{10}$ ____________

Change the following improper fractions to proper fractions.

101. $\frac{10}{5}$ ____________

102. $\frac{36}{9}$ ____________

103. $\frac{7}{5}$ ____________

104. $\frac{12}{3}$ ____________

105. $\frac{45}{5}$ ____________

106. $\frac{16}{12}$ ____________

107. $\frac{7}{6}$ ____________

108. $\frac{90}{15}$ ____________

109. $\frac{30}{2}$ ____________

110. $\frac{3}{2}$ ____________

Find least common multiples of the following sets of numbers.

111. 12, 4 ____________

112. 9, 3 ____________

113. 14, 2 ____________

114. 20, 4 ____________

115. 2, 10 ____________

116. 15, 50 ____________

117. 49, 7 ____________

118. 4, 6 ____________

119. 8, 2 ____________

120. 32, 8 ____________

Find the least common denominator in the following sets of fractions.

121. $\frac{1}{4}, \frac{1}{6}$ ____________

122. $\frac{3}{12}, \frac{4}{16}$ ____________

123. $\frac{2}{3}, \frac{4}{8}$ ____________

124. $\frac{15}{16}, \frac{2}{3}$ ____________

125. $\frac{3}{4}, \frac{4}{5}$ ____________

126. $\frac{6}{8}, \frac{3}{9}$ ____________

127. $\frac{12}{15}, \frac{3}{8}$ ____________

128. $\frac{2}{3}, \frac{6}{8}, \frac{4}{9}$ ____________

129. $\frac{1}{2}, \frac{2}{3}, \frac{6}{8}$ ____________

130. $\frac{3}{12}, \frac{5}{24}, \frac{2}{3}$ ____________

Add the following fractions with uncommon denominators.

131. $\frac{3}{12} + \frac{2}{3} =$ ____________

132. $\frac{3}{4} + \frac{6}{8} =$ ____________

133. $\frac{1}{2} + \frac{6}{7} =$ ____________

134. $\frac{4}{5} + \frac{1}{3} =$ ____________

135. $\frac{3}{8} + \frac{7}{16} =$ ____________

136. $\frac{4}{9} + \frac{2}{3} =$ ____________

137. $\frac{6}{12} + \frac{5}{9} =$ ____________

138. $\frac{2}{5} + \frac{7}{8} =$ ____________

139. $\frac{3}{7} + \frac{4}{5} =$ ____________

140. $\frac{6}{9} + \frac{2}{3} + \frac{1}{2} =$ ____________

Subtract the following fractions with uncommon denominators.

141. $\frac{2}{3} - \frac{1}{8} =$ ________________

142. $\frac{5}{6} - \frac{3}{8} =$ ________________

143. $\frac{1}{2} - \frac{1}{3} =$ ________________

144. $\frac{3}{4} - \frac{1}{6} =$ ________________

145. $\frac{7}{16} - \frac{8}{32} =$ ________________

146. $\frac{4}{6} - \frac{1}{3} =$ ________________

147. $\frac{7}{9} - \frac{2}{4} =$ ________________

148. $\frac{45}{50} - \frac{1}{3} =$ ________________

149. $\frac{12}{24} - \frac{3}{8} =$ ________________

150. $\frac{7}{8} - \frac{2}{16} =$ ________________

Subtract the following using borrowing.

151. $2 - \frac{2}{8} =$ ________________

152. $4\frac{1}{3} - \frac{2}{3} =$ ________________

153. $2\frac{1}{16} - 1\frac{3}{16} =$ ________________

154. $4\frac{1}{5} - \frac{4}{5} =$ ________________

155. $3\frac{6}{8} - 1\frac{7}{8} =$ ________________

156. $3\frac{1}{4} - 1\frac{3}{4} =$ ________________

157. $4\frac{12}{16} - \frac{15}{16} =$ ________________

158. $2\frac{1}{2} - \frac{3}{4} =$ ________________

159. $3\frac{1}{4} - 1\frac{1}{2} =$ ________________

160. $4\frac{3}{5} - 2\frac{4}{5} =$ ________________

Change the following mixed numbers to improper fractions.

161. $1\frac{1}{8}$ ________________

162. $3\frac{6}{9}$ ________________

163. $3\frac{1}{2}$ ________________

164. $12\frac{3}{4}$ ________________

165. $2\frac{5}{8}$ ________________

166. $2\frac{1}{5}$ ________________

167. $4\frac{5}{6}$ ________________

168. $1\frac{12}{16}$ ________________

169. $4\frac{1}{12}$ ________________

170. $3\frac{3}{4}$ ________________

Find the product of each of the following.

171. $\frac{3}{4} \times \frac{2}{3} =$ ________________

172. $\frac{1}{2} \times \frac{5}{6} =$ ________________

173. $\frac{3}{8} \times \frac{4}{5} =$ ________________

174. $\frac{5}{9} \times \frac{3}{4} =$ ________________

175. $\frac{12}{16} \times \frac{7}{8} =$ ________________

176. $\frac{2}{5} \times \frac{7}{8} =$ ________________

177. $\frac{1}{4} \times \frac{8}{9} =$ ________________

178. $\frac{2}{3} \times \frac{6}{18} =$ ________________

179. $\frac{4}{5} \times \frac{7}{8} =$ ________________

180. $\frac{2}{3} \times \frac{9}{8} =$ ________________

181. $\frac{2}{3} \times 12 =$ ________________

182. $\frac{3}{4} \times 2 =$ ________________

183. $3 \times \frac{15}{16} =$ ________________

184. $2\frac{1}{3} \times \frac{3}{4} =$ ________________

185. $\frac{3}{8} \times 1\frac{7}{8} =$ ________________

186. $\frac{4}{5} \times 2\frac{1}{4} =$ ________________

187. $\frac{5}{16} \times 8 =$ ________________

188. $12\frac{1}{8} \times 3\frac{1}{2} =$ ________________

189. $2\frac{2}{5} \times \frac{3}{5} =$ ________________

190. $1\frac{1}{2} \times 2\frac{3}{4} =$ ____________________

Find the quotient for each of the following.

191. $\frac{12}{16} \div \frac{2}{3} =$ ____________________

192. $\frac{1}{2} \div \frac{1}{3} =$ ____________________

193. $\frac{5}{6} \div \frac{7}{16} =$ ____________________

194. $\frac{3}{8} \div \frac{1}{5} =$ ____________________

195. $\frac{7}{8} \div \frac{2}{3} =$ ____________________

196. $\frac{14}{15} \div \frac{2}{3} =$ ____________________

197. $1\frac{2}{3} \div \frac{1}{8} =$ ____________________

198. $2\frac{4}{5} \div \frac{3}{4} =$ ____________________

199. $3\frac{1}{3} \div \frac{2}{3} =$ ____________________

200. $2\frac{1}{8} \div 1\frac{1}{16} =$ ____________________

INTRODUCTION

As a health care provider, you may see and use fractions on a daily basis. Whether you are preparing medication dosages for patients in an emergency department or measuring height and weight of residents in an extended care facility, the ability to understand fractions will help make your job easier.

Objective

6.1 Define fractions.

A **fraction** represents a part of a whole. For example, one-half of a pie is shown as $\frac{1}{2}$ and one-eighth of a pizza is shown as $\frac{1}{8}$. Fractions also provide a way to divide items, as shown in the following example.

Example

Five friends decide to split a pizza. If the pizza is divided into 10 equal slices, each of the 5 friends will get an equal share of two slices, as illustrated in Figure 6-1. Have you ever thought of using fractions in everyday activities like ordering pizza?

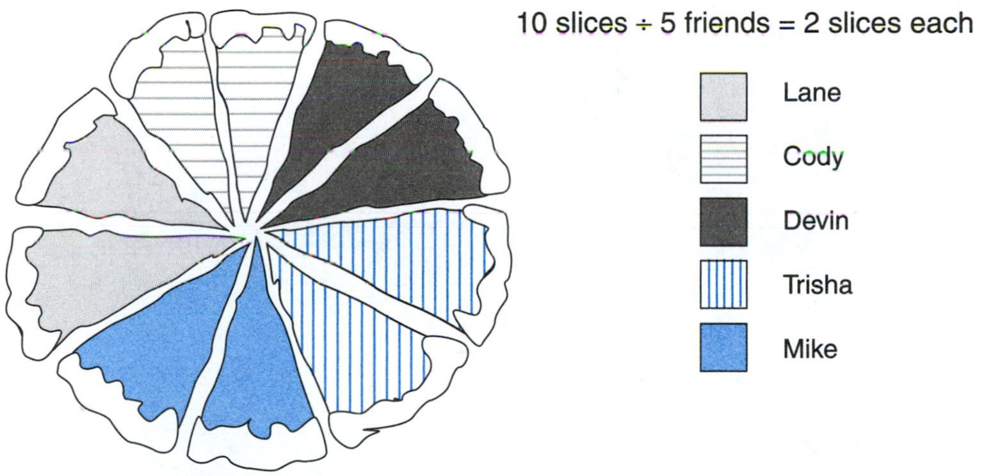

FIGURE 6-1 We use fractions daily, in such simple tasks as ordering pizza.

Objective

6.2 Explain advantages of using fractions.

As illustrated in the previous example, we utilize fractions in our everyday activities. Fractions help us to divide items into equal and unequal parts.

For example, a pie may be divided into 6 equal slices.

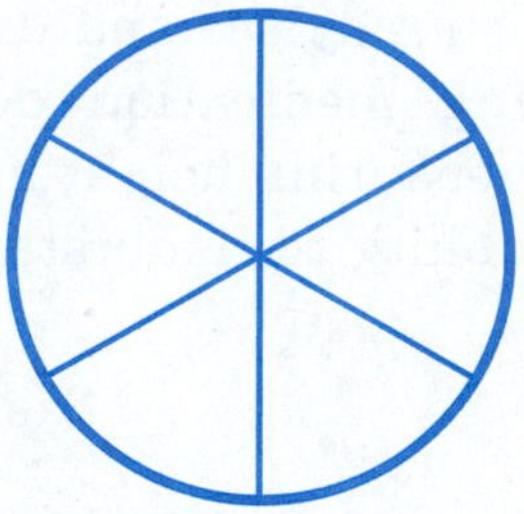

Alternately, one-half of the pie may be divided into three equal slices and the other half may be divided into four equal slices.

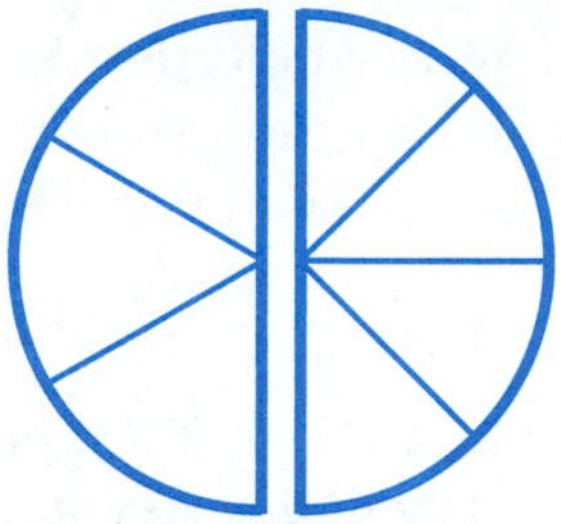

Regardless of how we decide to divide an item, fractions help to accomplish the task. See how many other items you can think of that we divide using fractions.

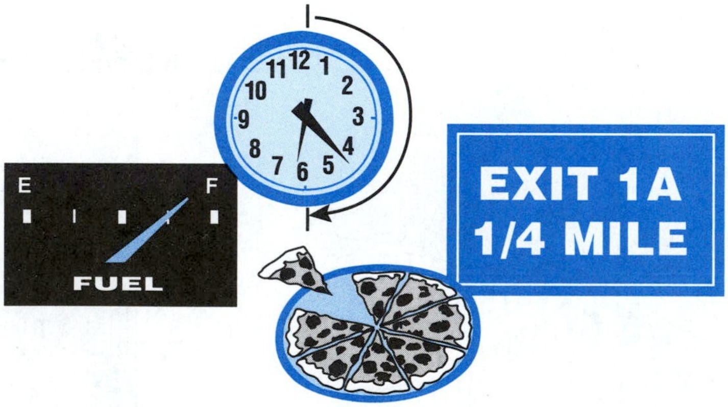

Objective

6.3 Find the numerator.

A **numerator** identifies the number of parts represented in the fraction. It is shown as the top number in the fraction.

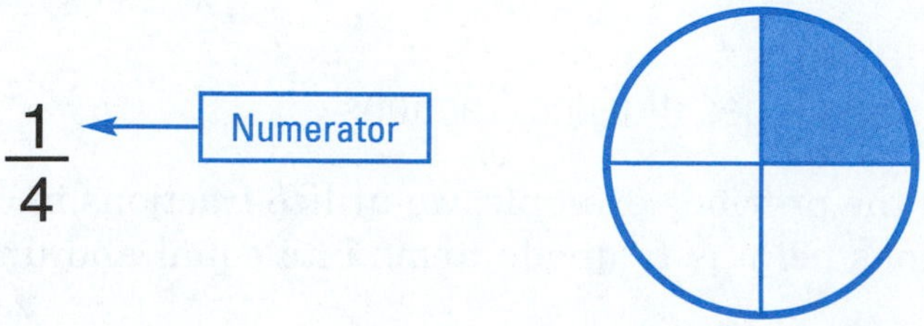

SKILL SHARPENER

Circle the numerator in the following fractions.

1. $\frac{1}{2}$
2. $\frac{4}{5}$
3. $\frac{12}{32}$
4. $\frac{6}{7}$
5. $\frac{9}{10}$
6. $\frac{12}{15}$
7. $\frac{3}{4}$
8. $\frac{8}{12}$
9. $\frac{10}{12}$
10. $\frac{5}{9}$

Objective

6.4 Find the denominator.

A **denominator** represents the number of parts into which an item is divided. For example, if the number below the line (denominator) is 2, the item is divided into 2 equal parts. If the denominator is 12, the item is divided into 12 equal parts.

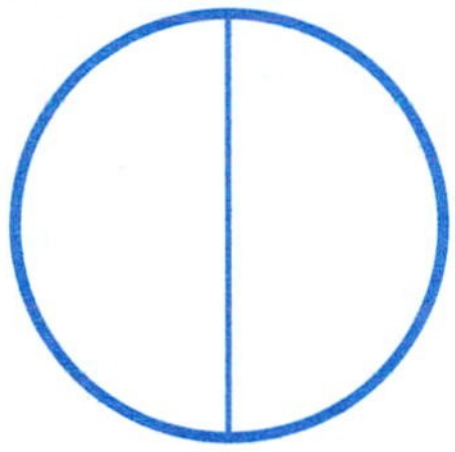

Denominator is 2

$\frac{}{2}$

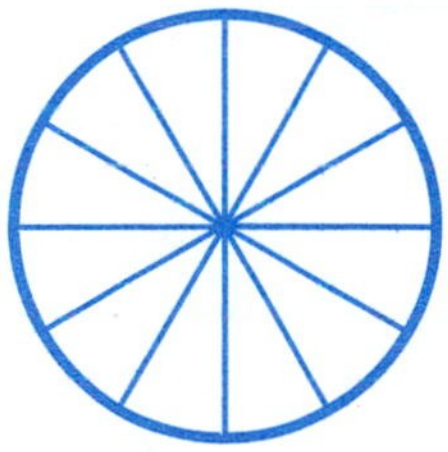

Denominator is 12

$\frac{}{12}$

SKILL SHARPENER

Circle the denominator in the following fractions.

1. $\frac{3}{4}$
2. $\frac{9}{16}$
3. $\frac{1}{2}$
4. $\frac{5}{8}$
5. $\frac{17}{32}$
6. $\frac{4}{7}$
7. $\frac{3}{8}$
8. $\frac{9}{16}$
9. $\frac{22}{100}$
10. $\frac{56}{9}$

Objective

6.5 Order fractions.

It is important to understand the value of fractions. Since the value of a fraction depends on both the numerator and denominator, you must consider both when determining the value of a fraction. Later, you will learn to find common denominators of fractions. This will make it easy to order fractions. For now, however, a simpler approach will help you begin to visualize fractions as part of a whole, rather than just a number on paper.

Example

Order the following fractions from lowest to highest, using the graphic representation of a pie to assist you. You may choose, instead, to convert each fraction to a decimal by dividing the numerator by the denominator. Then compare the decimals as demonstrated in Objective 5.4.

$\frac{1}{2}$ $\frac{1}{8}$ $\frac{1}{3}$ $\frac{2}{5}$

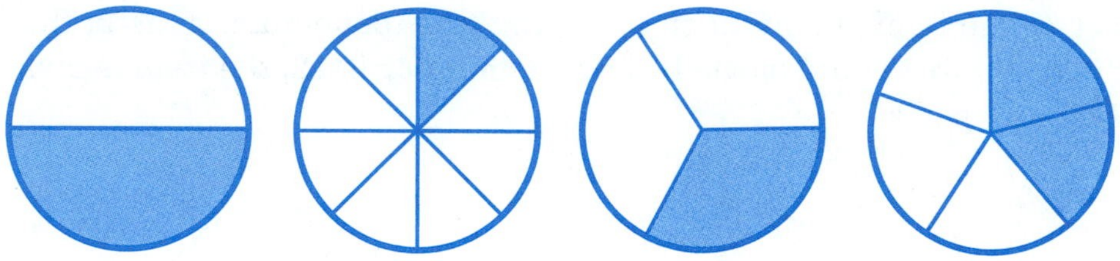

Compare the fractions using the graphic representation of the pies.

$\frac{1}{8}$ $\frac{1}{3}$ $\frac{2}{5}$ $\frac{1}{2}$

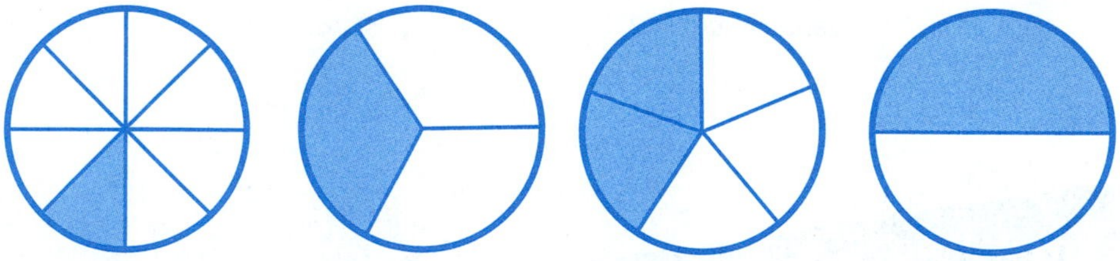

SKILL SHARPENER

Order the following fractions from smallest to largest.

1. $\frac{2}{3}$ $\frac{5}{8}$ $\frac{2}{5}$ ____________________

2. $\frac{2}{8}$ $\frac{1}{5}$ $\frac{6}{8}$ ____________________

3. $\frac{1}{2}$ $\frac{3}{4}$ $\frac{1}{5}$ ____________________

4. $\frac{1}{3}$ $\frac{2}{3}$ $\frac{1}{5}$ __________

5. $\frac{3}{6}$ $\frac{2}{3}$ $\frac{1}{5}$ __________

6. $\frac{3}{8}$ $\frac{1}{4}$ $\frac{1}{8}$ __________

7. $\frac{2}{6}$ $\frac{2}{3}$ $\frac{1}{8}$ __________

8. $\frac{4}{5}$ $\frac{3}{9}$ $\frac{2}{3}$ __________

9. $\frac{6}{7}$ $\frac{8}{9}$ $\frac{7}{8}$ __________

10. $\frac{1}{2}$ $\frac{5}{6}$ $\frac{3}{4}$ __________

Objective

6.6 Add fractions with common denominators.

There are times when fractions must be added. This is easily done when the fractions share **common denominators** or denominators that are the same. To find the sum of two or more fractions with common denominators, add the numerators. The denominator does not change. Write the sum of the numerators over the common denominator to reveal the solution. When the solution reveals an improper fraction, convert to a proper fraction or mixed number as illustrated in Objective 6.17.

The problem:

$$\frac{1}{8} + \frac{3}{8} = \_\_\_$$

Set up as:

$$\frac{1}{8} + \frac{3}{8} = \_\_\_$$

Add.

$$\frac{1+3}{8\quad 8} = \frac{4}{8}$$

Solution: $\frac{1}{8} + \frac{3}{8} = \frac{4}{8}$

SKILL SHARPENER

Add the following fractions.

1. $\frac{4}{5} + \frac{3}{5} =$ __________

2. $\frac{2}{3} + \frac{2}{3} =$ __________

3. $\frac{12}{16} + \frac{2}{16} =$ ______

4. $\frac{2}{6} + \frac{1}{6} =$ ______

5. $\frac{2}{9} + \frac{3}{9} =$ ______

6. $\frac{3}{8} + \frac{1}{8} =$ ______

7. $\frac{7}{8} + \frac{2}{8} =$ ______

8. $\frac{1}{7} + \frac{3}{7} =$ ______

9. $\frac{12}{50} + \frac{33}{50} =$ ______

10. $\frac{2}{25} + \frac{22}{25} =$ ______

Objective

6.7 Subtract fractions with common denominators.

To subtract fractions that share a common denominator, simply subtract the numerators. The denominator does not change. When solutions contain improper fractions, convert to proper fractions or mixed numbers as illustrated in Objective 6.17.

The problem:

$$\frac{9}{16} - \frac{3}{16} = \_\_\_\_$$

Set up as:

$$\frac{9}{16} - \frac{3}{16} = \_\_\_\_$$

Subtract.

$$\frac{9 - 3}{16 \quad 16} = \frac{6}{16}$$

Solution: $\frac{9}{16} - \frac{3}{16} = \frac{6}{16}$

SKILL SHARPENER

Subtract the following fractions.

1. $\frac{3}{4} - \frac{1}{4} =$ ________________

2. $\frac{9}{18} - \frac{3}{18} =$ ________________

3. $\frac{2}{3} - \frac{1}{3} =$ ________________

4. $\frac{9}{12} - \frac{4}{12} =$ ________________

5. $\frac{40}{50} - \frac{13}{50} =$ ________________

6. $\frac{12}{16} - \frac{3}{16} =$ ________________

7. $\frac{24}{100} - \frac{6}{100} =$ ________________

8. $\frac{7}{80} - \frac{2}{80} =$ ________________

9. $\frac{300}{1{,}200} - \frac{25}{1{,}200} =$ ________________

10. $\frac{7}{8} - \frac{5}{8} =$ ________________

Objective

6.8 Define mixed number.

A **mixed number** is a combination of a whole number and a fraction. As you will see, it is sometimes necessary to convert mixed numbers to improper fractions.

Objective

6.9 Add mixed numbers with common denominators.

To add mixed numbers with common denominators, first add the numerators of the fractions. The denominator will not change. If the sum of the numerators is greater than the denominator, convert the fraction to a mixed number. Then add the whole numbers and, if applicable, add the whole number of the mixed number.

The problem:

$$1\frac{1}{3} + 2\frac{1}{3} = \_\_\_\_$$

Set up as:

$$1\frac{1}{3} + 2\frac{1}{3} = \_\_\_\_$$

Add fractions.

$$\frac{1}{3} + \frac{1}{3} = \frac{2}{3}$$

Add whole numbers.

$$1 + 2 = 3$$

Combine.

$$3\frac{2}{3}$$

Solution: $1\frac{1}{3} + 2\frac{1}{3} = 3\frac{2}{3}$

SKILL SHARPENER

Add the following fractions.

1. $1\frac{2}{5} + 2\frac{1}{5} =$ ________________
2. $2\frac{6}{9} + 1\frac{1}{9} =$ ________________
3. $5\frac{1}{12} + 1\frac{5}{12} =$ ________________
4. $3\frac{2}{8} + 1\frac{5}{8} =$ ________________
5. $1\frac{13}{50} + 2\frac{2}{50} =$ ________________
6. $2\frac{3}{24} + 1\frac{6}{24} =$ ________________
7. $4\frac{5}{8} + 3\frac{1}{8} =$ ________________
8. $1\frac{3}{7} + 2\frac{1}{7} =$ ________________
9. $2\frac{1}{20} + 1\frac{1}{20} =$ ________________
10. $3\frac{15}{16} + 1\frac{2}{16} =$ ________________

Objective

6.10 Subtract mixed numbers with common denominators.

When subtracting mixed numbers with common denominators, first subtract the numerators of the fractions. If necessary, you may borrow from the whole number. Then subtract the whole numbers. The combination of the differences is your solution. You may also convert the mixed numbers to improper fractions as explained in Objective 6.24. Then subtract and convert the difference to a proper fraction or mixed number.

The problem:

$$3\frac{9}{16} - 1\frac{4}{16} = \_\_\_\_$$

Set up as:

$$3\frac{9}{16} - 1\frac{4}{16} = \_\_\_\_$$

Subtract fractions.

$$\frac{9}{16} - \frac{4}{16} = \frac{5}{16}$$

Subtract whole numbers.

$$3 - 1 = 2$$

Combine.

$$2\frac{5}{16}$$

Solution: $3\frac{9}{16} - 1\frac{4}{16} = 2\frac{5}{16}$

SKILL SHARPENER

Find the difference.

1. $1\frac{3}{4} - \frac{1}{4} =$ ________________

2. $5\frac{5}{6} - 1\frac{2}{6} =$ ________________

3. $3\frac{5}{24} - 1\frac{3}{24} =$ ________________

4. $2\frac{6}{8} - 1\frac{1}{8} =$ ________________

5. $1\frac{9}{10} - \frac{3}{10} =$ ________________

6. $11\frac{15}{16} - 5\frac{1}{16} =$ ______________________

7. $3\frac{4}{9} - 1\frac{1}{9} =$ ______________________

8. $3\frac{4}{11} - 1\frac{3}{11} =$ ______________________

9. $5\frac{15}{16} - 2\frac{12}{16} =$ ______________________

10. $9\frac{30}{100} - 6\frac{10}{100} =$ ______________________

Objective

6.11 Define factors.

Factors are pairs of numbers that, when multiplied, form a certain product. Factors of a number are found by using multiplication to determine every combination of that number.

Example

To find the factors of 16, determine every possible combination of 16 using multiplication.

$1 \times 16 = 16$
$2 \times 8 = 16$
$4 \times 4 = 16$

Factors of 16 are 1, 2, 4, 8, and 16.

Later, this skill will be used to perform other operations.

SKILL SHARPENER

Find the factors of the following numbers.

1. 8 ______________________

2. 9 ______________________

3. 12 ______________________

4. 18 ____________________

5. 24 ____________________

6. 20 ____________________

7. 10 ____________________

8. 6 ____________________

9. 14 ____________________

10. 22 ____________________

Objective

6.12 Find common factors.

A **common factor** is a factor that belongs to two or more numbers. To find the common factor(s) of two numbers, first find the factors for each number.

The problem:

Find factors of 8 and 12.

Find all the ways you can multiply to produce 8 and 12.

8	12
$1 \times 8 = 8$	$1 \times 12 = 12$
$2 \times 4 = 8$	$2 \times 6 = 12$
	$3 \times 4 = 12$

Now find the common factors.

8	12
$1 \times 8 = 8$	$1 \times 12 = 12$
$2 \times 4 = 8$	$2 \times 6 = 12$
	$3 \times 4 = 12$

Solution: Common factors of 8 and 12 are 1, 2, and 4.

The factors common to both numbers are common factors. Common factors in this set are 1, 2, and 4. Factors uncommon to a set of numbers are **uncommon factors**. The uncommon factors in this set are 3, 6, 8, and 12.

SKILL SHARPENER

Find common factors for the following sets of numbers.

1. 12, 16 ______________________
2. 8, 12 ______________________
3. 10, 15 ______________________
4. 24, 12 ______________________
5. 3, 8 ______________________
6. 5, 12 ______________________
7. 6, 9, 12 ______________________
8. 16, 8, 24 ______________________
9. 18, 6, 9 ______________________
10. 9, 36, 6 ______________________

Objective

6.13 Find the greatest common factor.

The **greatest common factor (GCF)** is the largest factor that two or more numbers have in common. To find the greatest common factor, first find the common factors. Then find the largest factor that the two numbers have in common. This is the greatest common factor.

In the earlier example, we found that common factors for 8 and 12 are 1, 2, and 4. Therefore, the greatest common factor for 8 and 12 is 4.

SKILL SHARPENER

Find the greatest common factor for the following sets of numbers.

1. 6, 9 __________

2. 12, 20 __________

3. 3, 12 __________

4. 9, 6 __________

5. 2, 3, 9 __________

6. 12, 24 __________

7. 5, 12 __________

8. 4, 12, 9 __________

9. 3, 5, 9 __________

10. 15, 3, 5 __________

Objective

6.14 Reduce fractions.

To make fractions clearer, reduce them to their lowest terms by finding the greatest common factor of the numerator and denominator. Divide both the numerator and denominator by their greatest common factor. The result is a reduced fraction.

To reduce $\frac{4}{6}$ to its lowest terms:

Find the factors of the numerator and denominator.

4	6
$1 \times 4 = 4$	$1 \times 6 = 6$
$2 \times 2 = 4$	$2 \times 3 = 6$

Find the GCF.

The GCF is 2.

Divide the numerator and denominator by the GCF to reduce the fraction to its lowest terms.

$$\frac{4 \div 2}{6 \div 2} = \frac{2}{3}$$

SKILL SHARPENER

Reduce the following fractions to their lowest terms.

1. $\frac{6}{8}$ ____________________
2. $\frac{5}{25}$ ____________________
3. $\frac{9}{81}$ ____________________
4. $\frac{6}{9}$ ____________________
5. $\frac{3}{6}$ ____________________
6. $\frac{2}{8}$ ____________________
7. $\frac{10}{20}$ ____________________
8. $\frac{11}{33}$ ____________________
9. $\frac{24}{48}$ ____________________
10. $\frac{3}{9}$ ____________________

Objective

6.15 Define proper fraction.

A **proper fraction** is one in which the denominator is greater than the numerator.

Proper fraction:

$$\frac{9}{16}$$

Numerator (**smaller**)
Denominator (**larger**)

SKILL SHARPENER

Determine if the following fractions are proper by placing **P** beside those that are proper and **I** (for improper) beside those that are not proper.

1. $\frac{3}{8}$ ________
2. $\frac{7}{16}$ ________
3. $\frac{9}{8}$ ________
4. $\frac{4}{3}$ ________
5. $\frac{12}{15}$ ________
6. $\frac{11}{16}$ ________
7. $\frac{90}{12}$ ________
8. $\frac{33}{2}$ ________
9. $\frac{12}{45}$ ________
10. $\frac{1}{25}$ ________

Objective

6.16 Define improper fraction.

An **improper fraction** is one in which the numerator is greater than the denominator. Improper fractions may be changed to proper fractions or mixed numbers to make them easier to read.

Improper fraction:

$\frac{12}{10}$ Numerator (**larger**) / Denominator (**smaller**)

SKILL SHARPENER

Place **P** beside the following fractions that are proper and **I** next to those that are improper.

1. $\frac{2}{4}$ ________
2. $\frac{9}{6}$ ________
3. $\frac{5}{4}$ ________
4. $\frac{15}{16}$ ________
5. $\frac{6}{9}$ ________
6. $\frac{12}{3}$ ________
7. $\frac{4}{8}$ ________
8. $\frac{2}{3}$ ________
9. $\frac{10}{2}$ ________
10. $\frac{6}{5}$ ________

Objective

6.17 Change improper fractions to proper fractions.

To change improper fractions to proper fractions, divide the denominator into the numerator. The result is a proper fraction that may or may not need to be reduced.

The problem:

Convert the improper fraction $\frac{23}{16}$ to a proper fraction.

Divide the denominator into the numerator.

$$23 \div 16 = \_\_\_\_$$

Set up as:

$$16\,\overline{)\,23}$$

Divide.

$$\begin{array}{r} 1 \\ 16\,\overline{)\,23} \\ \underline{16} \\ 7 \end{array}$$

Solution: $1\frac{7}{16}$

$$\begin{array}{r} 1 \\ 16\,\overline{)\,23} \\ \underline{16} \\ 7 \end{array}$$

Denominator → 16; Whole number ← 1; Numerator ← 7

SKILL SHARPENER

Change the following improper fractions to proper fractions or mixed numbers.

1. $\frac{9}{8}$ ________________

2. $\frac{15}{5}$ ________________

3. $\frac{12}{3}$ ________________

4. $\frac{12}{7}$ ________________

5. $\frac{6}{4}$ ______________________

6. $\frac{6}{3}$ ______________________

7. $\frac{8}{2}$ ______________________

8. $\frac{15}{4}$ ______________________

9. $\frac{19}{3}$ ______________________

10. $\frac{22}{12}$ ______________________

Objective

6.18 Define multiple.

A **multiple** of a number is the product of a whole number and another whole number.

Example

Multiples of **2** are 2, 4, 6, 8, 10, 12, 14, 16, 18, 20, 22, 24, and so on.

Multiples of **3** are 3, 6, 9, 12, 15, 18, 21, 24, 27, 30, 33, 36, and so on.

SKILL SHARPENER

List some multiples of each of the following numbers.

1. 4 ______________________

2. 5 ______________________

3. 6 ______________________

4. 7 ______________________________

5. 8 ______________________________

Objective

6.19 Define least common multiple.

The **least common multiple** is the smallest multiple that is shared by two or more numbers.

Example

Multiples of **2** are 2, 4, 6, 8, 10, 12, 14, 16, 18, 20, 22, 24, and so on.

Multiples of **3** are 3, 6, 9, 12, 15, 18, 21, 24, 27, 30, 33, 36, and so on.

Common multiples of **2** and **3** are 6, 12, 18, 24.

The least common multiple is 6.

SKILL SHARPENER

Find the least common multiples of the following.

1. 2, 4 ______________________________

2. 3, 6 ______________________________

3. 4, 5 ______________________________

4. 12, 3 ______________________________

5. 7, 2 ______________________________

6. 8, 3 ______________________________

7. 9, 2 ________________________________

8. 10, 20, 4 ________________________________

9. 9, 12, 4 ________________________________

10. 2, 6, 8 ________________________________

Objective

6.20 Find the least common denominator.

The **least common denominator (LCD)** is the lowest number into which all the denominators in a set can be divided. To find the least common denominator, find the least common multiple of each of the denominators in the set.

The problem:

Find the least common denominator of $\frac{1}{4}$, $\frac{1}{3}$, and $\frac{1}{6}$.

Find the multiples of each denominator.

4, 8, 12, 16, 20, 24, and so on.

3, 6, 9, 12, 15, 18, 21, and so on.

6, 12, 18, 24, 30, and so on.

Find least common multiple (LCM).

4, 8, **12**, 16, 20, 24, and so on.

LCM → 3, 6, 9, **12**, 15, 18, 21, and so on.

6, **12**, 18, 24, 30, and so on.

Solution: The least common multiple is 12; therefore, the LCD is 12.

SKILL SHARPENER

Find the least common denominator for each of the following sets of fractions.

1. $\frac{2}{3}$ $\frac{5}{6}$ __________

2. $\frac{1}{2}$ $\frac{3}{4}$ __________

3. $\frac{7}{8}$ $\frac{7}{16}$ __________

4. $\frac{3}{4}$ $\frac{4}{5}$ __________

5. $\frac{8}{10}$ $\frac{12}{20}$ __________

6. $\frac{3}{8}$ $\frac{7}{16}$ __________

7. $\frac{7}{8}$ $\frac{1}{4}$ $\frac{2}{3}$ __________

8. $\frac{4}{5}$ $\frac{3}{10}$ __________

9. $\frac{2}{3}$ $\frac{3}{4}$ $\frac{4}{5}$ __________

10. $\frac{1}{2}$ $\frac{6}{8}$ $\frac{3}{4}$ __________

Objective

6.21 Add fractions with uncommon denominators.

To add fractions with **uncommon denominators**, first find the least common denominator. Next, convert each fraction to a fraction utilizing the least common denominator. Then add the numerators and reduce as necessary.

The problem:

Add the following fractions with uncommon denominators:

$$\frac{3}{4} + \frac{1}{3} = \_\_\_\_$$

Find the LCM and the LCD.

4, 8, 12, 16, 20, and so on.

3, 6, 9, 12, 15, and so on.

The LCM is 12, so the LCD will be 12.

Now change the denominators in both fractions to the LCD.

$$\frac{3}{4} + \frac{1}{3} = \_\_\_\_$$

$$\frac{\quad}{12} + \frac{\quad}{12} = \_\_\_\_$$

Multiply each numerator by the number of times the original denominators go into the LCD.

$$\frac{3}{4} + \frac{1}{3}$$

$4 \times 3 = 12$ | $\times 3$ | $\times 4$ | $3 \times 4 = 12$

$$\frac{\quad}{12} + \frac{\quad}{12}$$

Now multiply the original numerators by the shaded factors to determine new numerators.

$3 \times 3 = 9$ → $\frac{9}{12} + \frac{4}{12}$ ← $1 \times 4 = 4$

Add.

$$\frac{9}{12} + \frac{4}{12} = \frac{13}{12}$$

Solution: $\frac{3}{4} + \frac{1}{3} = \frac{13}{12}$ or $1\frac{1}{12}$

SKILL SHARPENER

Add the following fractions with uncommon denominators.

1. $\frac{1}{3} + \frac{2}{4} =$ ______

2. $\frac{2}{3} + \frac{1}{2} =$ ______

3. $\frac{3}{4} + \frac{7}{8} =$ ______

4. $\frac{1}{2} + \frac{3}{8} =$ ______

5. $\frac{3}{9} + \frac{2}{3} =$ ______

6. $\frac{4}{5} + \frac{5}{6} =$ ______

7. $\frac{1}{4} + \frac{1}{16} =$ ______

8. $\frac{2}{5} + \frac{6}{10} =$ ______

9. $\frac{3}{8} + \frac{9}{16} =$ ______

10. $\frac{3}{10} + \frac{19}{20} + \frac{3}{5} =$ ______

Objective

6.22 Subtract fractions with uncommon denominators.

To subtract fractions with uncommon denominators, find the least common denominator. Next, convert each fraction to a fraction utilizing the least common denominator. Then subtract the numerators and reduce as necessary.

The problem:

$$\frac{1}{2} - \frac{1}{16} = \_\_\_\_$$

Find the LCM, which will also be the LCD.

2, 4, 6, 8, 10, 12, 14, 16, and so on.

16, 32, 48, 64, and so on.

Solution: The LCM is 16; therefore, the LCD is 16.

Now change the denominators in both fractions to the LCD.

$$\frac{1}{2} - \frac{1}{16} = \underline{\qquad}$$

$$\frac{\ }{16} - \frac{\ }{16} = \underline{\qquad}$$

Multiply each numerator by the number of times the original denominators go into the LCD.

$$\frac{1}{2} - \frac{1}{16}$$

2 × 8 = 16 | × 8 | × 1 | 16 × 1 = 16

$$\frac{\ }{16} - \frac{\ }{16}$$

Now multiply the original numerators by the shaded factors.

1 × 8 = 8 → $\frac{8}{16} - \frac{1}{16}$ ← 1 × 1 = 1

Subtract.

$$\frac{8}{16} - \frac{1}{16} = \frac{7}{16}$$

Solution: $\frac{1}{2} - \frac{1}{16} = \frac{7}{16}$

SKILL SHARPENER

Subtract the following fractions with uncommon denominators.

1. $\frac{2}{3} - \frac{1}{4} =$ ____________________

2. $\frac{12}{16} - \frac{1}{2} =$ ____________________

3. $\frac{4}{5} - \frac{1}{3} =$ ____________________

4. $\frac{7}{8} - \frac{3}{5} =$ ____________________

5. $\frac{9}{10} - \frac{2}{5} =$ ____________________

6. $\frac{3}{4} - \frac{1}{2} =$ ____________________

7. $\frac{9}{18} - \frac{1}{3} =$ ______________________

8. $\frac{8}{9} - \frac{3}{7} =$ ______________________

9. $\frac{5}{9} - \frac{3}{8} =$ ______________________

10. $\frac{7}{11} - \frac{1}{22} =$ ______________________

Objective

6.23 Use borrowing to subtract fractions.

When subtracting mixed numbers, it is sometimes necessary to borrow. If fractions have uncommon denominators, find the least common denominator before subtracting.

The problem:

$$5\frac{1}{3} - 2\frac{2}{3} = \_\_\_\_\_$$

Subtract fractions.

$$\frac{1}{3} - \frac{2}{3} = \_\_\_\_\_$$

Since you cannot subtract 2 from 1, you will have to borrow from the whole number 5.

$$\not{5}\frac{1}{3} - 2\frac{2}{3}$$

$$\downarrow$$

$$4\frac{4}{3} - 2\frac{2}{3}$$

Now subtract the fractions.

$$\frac{4}{3} - \frac{2}{3} = \frac{2}{3}$$

Subtract the whole numbers.

$$4 - 2 = 2$$

Combine.

$$2\frac{2}{3}$$

Solution: $5\frac{1}{3} - 2\frac{2}{3} = 2\frac{2}{3}$

Note: An alternate way to subtract this is to convert to improper fractions.

$$5\frac{1}{3} - 2\frac{2}{3} = \_\_\_\_\_$$

To convert, multiply the denominator by the whole number and add the numerator.

$$(3 \times 5) + 1 - (3 \times 2) + 2$$

$$15 + 1 \quad - \quad 6 + 2$$

$$\frac{16}{3} \quad - \quad \frac{8}{3} = \frac{8}{3}$$

Now convert back to a proper fraction by dividing the numerator by the denominator.

$$8 \div 3 = \_\_\_\_$$

$$3\overline{)8}\ \text{quotient } 2;\quad 8 - 6 = 2$$

Solution: $5\frac{1}{3} - 2\frac{2}{3} = 2\frac{2}{3}$

Now practice by solving this problem in which the denominators are different.

$$4\frac{1}{4} - 2\frac{3}{8} = \_\_\_\_$$

The problem: Subtract the following fractions with uncommon denominators:

$$4\frac{1}{4} - 2\frac{3}{8} = \_\_\_\_$$

Find the LCM and LCD.

4, 8, 12, 16, 20, and so on.

8, 16, 24, 32, 40, and so on.

Now change the denominators in both fractions to the LCD.

$$4\frac{1}{4} - 2\frac{3}{8} = \_\_\_\_$$

$$\frac{\ }{8} - \frac{\ }{8} = \_\_\_\_$$

Multiply each numerator by the number of times the original denominator goes into the LCD.

$$4\frac{1}{4} - 2\frac{3}{8}$$

4 × 2 = 8 | × 2 | × 1 | 8 × 1 = 8

$$4\frac{\ }{8} - 2\frac{\ }{8}$$

Now multiply the original numerators by the shaded factors.

1 × 2 = 2 → $4\frac{2}{8} - 2\frac{3}{8}$ ← 3 × 1 = 3

Subtract.

$$4\frac{2}{8} - 2\frac{3}{8} = \_\_\_\_$$

Borrow.

$$4\frac{2}{8} - 2\frac{3}{8} = \_\_\_\_\_$$

$$3\frac{10}{8} - 2\frac{3}{8} = \_\_\_\_\_$$

Subtract fractions.

$$\frac{10}{8} - \frac{3}{8} = \frac{7}{8}$$

Subtract whole numbers.

$$3 - 2 = 1$$

Combine.

$$1\frac{7}{8}$$

Solution: $4\frac{1}{4} - 2\frac{3}{8} = 1\frac{7}{8}$

Now figure this problem by converting to improper fractions. The result should be the same.

SKILL SHARPENER

Subtract the following fractions.

1. $4\frac{5}{7} - 1\frac{1}{7} =$ __________

2. $3\frac{1}{2} - 1\frac{1}{2} =$ __________

3. $7\frac{3}{4} - 3\frac{1}{4} =$ __________

4. $4\frac{3}{8} - \frac{1}{8} =$ __________

5. $3\frac{15}{16} - 1\frac{5}{16}$

6. $4\frac{3}{4} - 2\frac{7}{8}$

7. $5\frac{1}{2} - 2\frac{7}{8}$

8. $6\frac{7}{8} - \frac{11}{12}$

9. $2\frac{3}{5} - 1\frac{5}{8}$

10. $1\frac{2}{3} - \frac{9}{11}$

Objective

6.24 Change mixed numbers to improper fractions.

To change a mixed number to an improper fraction, multiply the denominator by the whole number and add the numerator. This is your new numerator. The denominator stays the same.

The problem:

Change $4\frac{3}{8}$ to an improper fraction.

Multiply the whole number and denominator.

$4 \times 8 = 32$

Add the numerator.

$32 + 3 = 35$

This is the new numerator. The denominator does not change.

Solution: $4\frac{3}{8} = \frac{35}{8}$

Note: Another way to set up the equation is:

(whole number × denominator)	+	numerator	=	______
(4 × 8)	+	3	=	______
32	+	3	=	35

SKILL SHARPENER

Change these mixed numbers to improper fractions.

1. $3\frac{2}{9}$ ____________________
2. $8\frac{5}{8}$ ____________________
3. $2\frac{3}{4}$ ____________________
4. $7\frac{2}{6}$ ____________________
5. $1\frac{3}{11}$ ____________________
6. $9\frac{34}{50}$ ____________________
7. $6\frac{9}{12}$ ____________________
8. $5\frac{5}{9}$ ____________________
9. $12\frac{6}{10}$ ____________________
10. $3\frac{1}{2}$ ____________________

Objective

6.25 Multiply fractions.

To multiply simple fractions, find the product of the numerators and the product of the denominators. Reduce if necessary.

The problem:

$$\frac{1}{3} \times \frac{2}{3} = \_\_\_\_$$

Set up as:

$$\frac{1 \times 2 =}{3 \times 3 =}$$

Multiply:

$$\frac{1 \times 2 = 2}{3 \times 3 = 9}$$

Solution: $\frac{1}{3} \times \frac{2}{3} = \frac{2}{9}$

SKILL SHARPENER

Find the products of the following fractions.

1. $\frac{2}{3} \times \frac{3}{4} =$ ________________

2. $\frac{1}{8} \times \frac{2}{3} =$ ________________

3. $\frac{4}{5} \times \frac{7}{8} =$ ________________

4. $\frac{1}{2} \times \frac{5}{9} =$ ________________

5. $\frac{2}{6} \times \frac{3}{4} =$ ________________

6. $\frac{4}{8} \times \frac{1}{5} =$ ________________

7. $\frac{3}{8} \times \frac{1}{2} =$ ________________

8. $\frac{5}{8} \times \frac{2}{6} =$ ________________

9. $\frac{7}{9} \times \frac{1}{10} =$ ________________

10. $\frac{3}{5} \times \frac{2}{7} =$ ________________

Objective

6.26 Multiply fractions using canceling.

To utilize **canceling** to find the product of two fractions, set the equation up as follows.

The problem:

$$\frac{3}{8} \times \frac{4}{12} = \underline{\hspace{2em}}$$

Cancel by determining if any numerator or denominator is divisible by another.

$$\frac{3}{8} \times \frac{4}{12} = \underline{\hspace{2em}}$$

Since 4 goes into 8 twice, replace the 8 with 2 and the 4 with 1:

$$_2\frac{3}{\not 8} \times \frac{\not 4^{\,1}}{12}$$

Since 3 goes into 12 four times, cancel the 3 and write 1 and replace the 12 with 4:

$$^1\frac{\not 3}{2} \times \frac{1}{\not 12}\,_4$$

We now have:

$$\frac{1}{2} \times \frac{1}{4} = \underline{\hspace{2em}}$$

Multiply.

$$\frac{1 \times 1 = 1}{2 \times 4 = 8}$$

Solution: $\frac{3}{8} \times \frac{4}{12} = \frac{1}{8}$

SKILL SHARPENER

Find the product using canceling.

1. $\frac{1}{6} \times \frac{2}{3} =$ ______
2. $\frac{3}{9} \times \frac{1}{3} =$ ______
3. $\frac{1}{2} \times \frac{4}{8} =$ ______
4. $\frac{3}{4} \times \frac{1}{6} =$ ______
5. $\frac{4}{7} \times \frac{5}{6} =$ ______

6. $\frac{3}{8} \times \frac{2}{6} =$ __________

7. $\frac{7}{9} \times \frac{3}{4} =$ __________

8. $\frac{5}{6} \times \frac{3}{4} =$ __________

9. $\frac{5}{15} \times \frac{1}{5} =$ __________

10. $\frac{4}{6} \times \frac{12}{16} =$ __________

Objective

6.27 Multiply fractions and whole numbers.

When multiplying fractions and whole numbers, first convert the whole number to an improper fraction. Multiply numerators and denominators. Then convert back to a proper fraction or mixed number.

The problem:

$$3 \times \frac{1}{8} = \_\_\_\_$$

Convert the whole number to an improper fraction by using a denominator of 1.

$$\frac{3}{1} \times \frac{1}{8} = \_\_\_\_$$

Multiply the numerators and denominators.

$$\frac{3 \times 1 = 3}{1 \times 8 = 8}$$

Solution: $3 \times \frac{1}{8} = \frac{3}{8}$

SKILL SHARPENER

Find the products.

1. $\frac{2}{3} \times 12 =$ __________

2. $3 \times \frac{1}{5} =$ __________

3. $4 \times \frac{4}{5} =$ __________

4. $2 \times \frac{5}{6} =$ __________

5. $\begin{array}{r} \frac{1}{2} \\ \times 10 \\ \hline \end{array}$

6. $\begin{array}{r} \frac{1}{3} \\ \times 5 \\ \hline \end{array}$

7. $\begin{array}{r} \frac{4}{6} \\ \times 9 \\ \hline \end{array}$

8. $\begin{array}{r} 3 \\ \times \frac{5}{9} \\ \hline \end{array}$

9. $\begin{array}{r} 9 \\ \times \frac{5}{16} \\ \hline \end{array}$

10. $\begin{array}{r} 5 \\ \times \frac{1}{9} \\ \hline \end{array}$

Objective

6.28 Multiply fractions and mixed numbers.

To multiply a fraction with a mixed number, convert the mixed number to an improper fraction. Then multiply to find the product of the numerators and the product of the denominators. Reduce to lowest terms.

The problem:

$$\frac{1}{5} \times 2\frac{1}{2} = \_\_\_\_\_$$

Convert the mixed number ($2\frac{1}{2}$) to an improper fraction.

Multiply the whole number by the denominator, then add the numerator.

(whole number × denominator)	+	numerator	=	_____
(2 × 2)	+	1	=	_____
4	+	1	=	5

The new numerator is 5. The denominator stays the same.

$$\frac{5}{2}$$

Set up as:

$$\frac{1}{5} \times \frac{5}{2} = \_\_\_\_\_$$

Multiply the numerators and denominators. In this case, you may use canceling to change both 5s to 1s.

Multiply

$$\frac{1 \times 5 = 5}{5 \times 2 = 10}$$

Cancel

$$\frac{1}{\cancel{5}_{1}} \times \frac{\cancel{5}^{1}}{2} = \frac{1}{2}$$

If necessary, reduce by finding the LCF.*

5	10
$1 \times 5 = 5$	$1 \times 10 = 10$
	$2 \times 5 = 10$

LCF is 5. Divide 5 into $\frac{5}{10}$.

$$\frac{5 \div 5}{10 \div 5} = \frac{1}{2}$$

Solution: $\frac{1}{5} \times 2\frac{1}{2} = \frac{1}{2}$

*By canceling, you eliminate one step (reducing).

SKILL SHARPENER

Find the product. Reduce to lowest terms.

1. $\frac{2}{3} \times 3\frac{1}{2}$

2. $\frac{3}{5} \times 2\frac{3}{4}$

3. $1\frac{3}{4} \times \frac{2}{5}$

4. $4\frac{5}{8} \times \frac{3}{16}$

5. $2\frac{1}{2} \times \frac{4}{5}$

6. $3\frac{1}{8} \times \frac{9}{10}$

7. $5\frac{3}{7} \times \frac{1}{11} =$ __________

8. $\frac{7}{8} \times 8\frac{3}{8} =$ __________

9. $\frac{6}{7} \times 3\frac{3}{9} =$ __________

10. $\frac{2}{5} \times 12\frac{4}{8} =$ __________

Objective

6.29 Divide fractions.

To divide fractions, convert any mixed numbers to improper fractions. Invert the divisor and multiply numerators and denominators.

The problem:

$$\frac{4}{9} \div \frac{1}{3} = \_\_\_\_$$

Invert divisor and change division symbol to multiplication.

$$\frac{4}{9} \times \frac{3}{1} = \_\_\_\_$$

Multiply numerators and denominators.

$$\frac{4 \times 3 = 12}{9 \times 1 = \ 9}$$

Reduce by dividing the product by the LCF.

12	9
1 × 12 = 12	1 × 9 = 9
2 × 6 = 12	**3** × 3 = 9
3 × 4 = 12	

LCF is 3.

$$\frac{12 \div 3 = 4}{9 \div 3 = 3}$$

OR

Multiply by canceling.

$$_{3}\frac{4}{\cancel{9}} \times \frac{\cancel{3}^{\,1}}{1}$$

Then multiply numerators and denominators.

$$_{3}\frac{4}{\cancel{9}} \times \frac{\cancel{3}^{\,1}}{1} = \frac{4}{3}$$

Convert to mixed number.

$$4 \div 3 = \_\_\_\_$$

$$3\overline{)4} \text{ quotient } 1,\quad 4 - 3 = 1$$

Denominator → 3

1 ← Whole number

1 ← Numerator

Solution: $\frac{4}{9} \div \frac{1}{3} = 1\frac{1}{3}$

SKILL SHARPENER

Divide the following fractions.

1. $\frac{3}{8} \div \frac{1}{4} =$ ______________________

2. $\frac{7}{8} \div \frac{2}{3} =$ ______________________

3. $\frac{16}{18} \div \frac{9}{12} =$ ______________________

4. $\frac{3}{4} \div \frac{1}{3} =$ ______________________

5. $\frac{2}{5} \overline{\big)\, \frac{8}{10}}$

6. $\frac{2}{3} \overline{\big)\, 1\frac{3}{8}}$

7. $\frac{1}{2} \overline{\big)\, 3\frac{2}{5}}$

8. $1\frac{7}{8} \overline{\big)\, 4\frac{1}{2}}$

9. $2\frac{6}{7} \overline{\big)\, 12\frac{5}{8}}$

10. $\frac{3}{4} \overline{\big)\, 2\frac{8}{10}}$

CONCLUSION

Fractions are used in many ways in the health care industry. Medication dosages, heights and weights, and many other measurements use fractions. The ability to add, subtract, multiply, and divide fractions will help you to better perform as a health care provider, thus providing better care to your patients.

REVIEW AND REFLECT

1. Why should fractions be reduced to their lowest terms?

2. Why is it important to understand how to find multiples?

3. Discuss several ways to use fractions in everyday life.

4. When should canceling be used to multiply fractions?

5. Why is borrowing sometimes used when subtracting fractions?

CHAPTER

7

Ratios and Proportions

LEARNING **OBJECTIVES**

After completing this chapter, the reader will be able to:

- **7.1** Define ratio.
- **7.2** Define proportion.
- **7.3** Determine if proportions are equal.
- **7.4** Solve for a missing component in a proportion.
- **7.5** Solve practical problems using proportions.

KEY **TERMS**

- extremes
- means
- proportion
- ratio
- terms

MATH IN THE REAL WORLD

"Ratios are used for medications like D50 (dextrose 50%) that must be diluted to D25 (dextrose 25%) for children. Additionally, we use proportions in calculating medication dosages."

Roger G. Wootten, AAS, EMT-Paramedic

SELF-ASSESSMENT **PRETEST**

Write the following ratios using colons. Reduce to lowest terms.

1. 7 patients out of 8 patients ____________

2. 3 ambulances out of 12 ambulances ____________

3. 33 surgeries out of 66 surgeries ____________

4. 9 prescriptions out of 27 prescriptions ____________

5. 20 days out of 30 days ____________

6. 3 physical therapists to 2 occupational therapists ____________

7. 1 RN to 3 CNAs ____________

8. 12 green stethoscopes to 48 blue stethoscopes ____________

9. 24 patients to 6 staff members ____________

10. 38 scheduled surgeries to 3 operating rooms ____________

Determine if the following proportions are equal.

11. 124 : 10 : : 1240 : 100 ____________

12. 90 : 15 : : 4 : 2 ____________

13. 4 : 1 : : 90 : 15 ____________

14. 75 : 19 : : 5 : 1 ____________

15. 100 : 10 : : 10 : 1 ____________

16. 25 : 5 : : 20 : 4 ____________

17. 25 : 5 : : 20 : 3 ____________

18. 150 : 50 : : 3 : 1 ____________

19. 48 : 84 : : 84 : 168 ____________

20. 365 : 12 : : 205 : 1 ____________

Solve for the missing component (x) in each of the following proportions.

21. 50 : 150 : : 1 : x ____________

22. 180 : x : : 12 : 24 ____________

23. 36 : 18 : : x : 9 ____________

24. x : 900 : : 300 : 1 ____________

25. 24 : 72 : : x : 6 ____________

26. 980 : 98 : : 7 : x ____________

27. x : 23 : : 49 : 46 ____________

28. 450 : 45 : : 10 : x ____________

29. 248 : 3 : : x : 4 ____________

30. 657 : x : : 757 : 100 ____________

Solve the following problems using proportions.

31. You are asked to administer 75 milligrams (mg) of Lidocaine. It is packaged 10 mg per 1 milliliter (mL). How many mL do you administer?

____

32. You have $1,238 of your total stock portfolio of $36,898 in international stocks. What percentage of your total stock portfolio is in international stocks?

____

33. The physician asks you to administer 5 mg of atenolol to Mrs. Jones. Atenolol is packaged 1 mg per 2 mL. How many mL will you administer to Mrs. Jones?

____

34. You are asked to administer 60 mg of furosemide to Mr. Genheim. The packaging you have on hand is 10 mg per mL in 4 mL ampules. How many ampules do you need?

____

35. If 1/5 of the light bulbs in your house are 40 watts and lower, and there are 60 bulbs in your house, what percentage of bulbs in your house are 40 watts and lower?

____

36. Your car gets 31 miles per gallon on the highway and 26 miles per gallon in the city. What percentage of mileage does your car get in the city compared to on the highway?

____

37. You need to administer naloxone to Ms. Reed. The order is for 0.6 mg intramuscularly. Naloxone is packaged 0.4 mg/mL in 1 mL vials. How many mL do you administer?

____

38. You have an adult patient that has second degree burns on approximately 2/3 of his anterior torso. Since you know that the entire anterior torso accounts for approximately 18% of total body surface area, determine what percentage of his total body surface area is burned.

____

39. Your teacher has developed a strange new grading system in which she requires that you attain at least 75% of the total points available to pass. You have obtained 1,132 points out of a possible 1,380. Did you pass the class?

____

40. Mrs. Reed's electrocardiogram reveals a QRS complex that is 30% wider than the normal limit of 0.12 seconds. How long is the QRS complex?

____

INTRODUCTION

Ratios and proportions are commonly used in health care and medicine to compare measurements. Many health care providers utilize ratios and proportions on a daily basis to solve a variety of equations and make comparisons between unlike items.

Objective

7.1 Define ratio.

As you have already learned, we can compare quantities in different ways. A **ratio** is a comparison of numbers by division. The numbers that are compared are called the **terms**, or components, of the ratio. For example, we can compare the number of blue stethoscopes to the number of black stethoscopes in Figure 7-1.

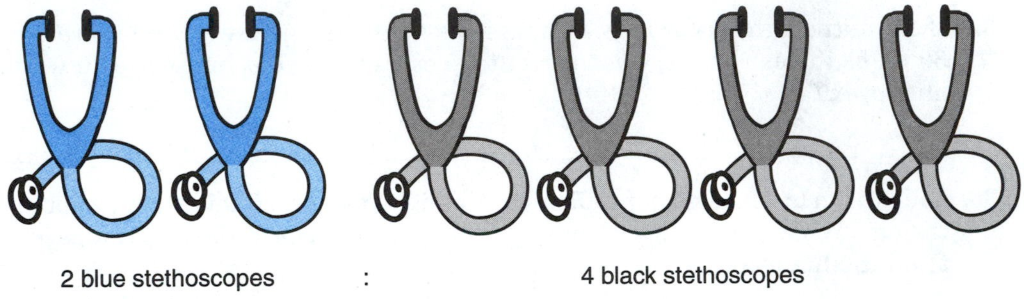

FIGURE 7-1 This ratio is expressed as 2:4.

There are two blue stethoscopes and four black stethoscopes. Therefore, the ratio is 2 to 4, which may also be expressed as 2:4 or 2/4.

There is another way to express this ratio by reducing to the lowest common denominator. The ratio of 1 to 2 is also correct. For every one blue stethoscope, there are two black stethoscopes. Generally speaking, reducing to the LCD is helpful, especially when dealing with large numbers. Ratios are helpful in that they allow you to compare both like measurements and unlike measurements.

Consider the following examples.

Example A

On the day shift in the local hospital, there are two physical therapists and six physical therapy assistants on duty. What is the ratio of physical therapists to physical therapy assistants? Are these measurements alike or unlike?

If you answered 1:3 or 2:6 you are correct. And, of course, a physical therapist is unlike a physical therapy assistant (though the two are both measured as people). This ratio, or comparison, made it simple to measure the comparison between the two.

Example B

As you have likely learned, 1 pound is equal to 2.2 kg. State the ratio involved. Are these measurements alike or unlike?

If you answered 1:2.2 you are correct. Again, the measurements are unlike in that you are comparing pounds to kilograms.

Objective

7.2 Define proportion.

A **proportion** is an equation that states that two ratios are equal. Proportions are set up as 1:2::2:4. This is read: 1 is to 2 as 2 is to 4. The middle components of the proportion are called the **means** and the end, or outside, components are called **extremes**.

Means

1 : 2 :: 2 : 4

Extremes

Objective

7.3 Determine if proportions are equal.

Comparing the product of the means to the product of the extremes determines if a proportion is equal. If the product of the means is equal to the product of the extremes, the proportion is said to be equal.

The problem: Determine if the proportion is equal:

1:2::2:4

Find the product of the means and the extremes.

Multiply the means: 1:2::2:4

$2 \times 2 = 4$

Multiply the extremes: 1:2::2:4

$1 \times 4 = 4$

Determine if means = extremes.

$4 = 4$

By multiplying the means ($2 \times 2 = 4$) and multiplying the extremes ($1 \times 4 = 4$) we can see that the products are equal.

Solution: The proportion, 1:2::2:4, is equal.

SKILL SHARPENER

Determine if the following proportions are equal.

1. 12:144::1:12 ____________________
2. 24:250::48:600 ____________________
3. 6:9::2:3 ____________________
4. 100:10::1000:100 ____________________
5. 230:10::23:1 ____________________
6. 10:23::1:230 ____________________
7. 234:43::23:4 ____________________
8. 231:1::462:2 ____________________
9. 231:1::243:2 ____________________
10. 450:9000::1:20 ____________________

Objective

7.4 Solve for a missing component in a proportion.

Often, one component of a proportion is unknown. Solve for the unknown component (x) as shown here.

The problem:

$$12 : x :: 6 : 1$$

Find the product of the means and the extremes.

Multiply the means: 12 : x :: 6 : 1

$$x \times 6 = 6x$$

Multiply the extremes: 12 : x :: 6 : 1

$$12 \times 1 = 12$$

Set up as:

$$6x = 12$$

To solve for x, divide each side by 6.

$6x \div 6 = 1x$ (or just x)

$12 \div 6 = 2$

$x = 2$

Solution: 12 : 2 :: 6 : 1

SKILL SHARPENER

Find the missing component (x) in each of the following proportions.

1. 12:6 :: x:12 ____________________
2. 20:x :: 1:10 ____________________
3. x:34 :: 34:2 ____________________
4. 2.5:1 :: 10:x ____________________
5. 100:3 :: x:900 ____________________
6. 4:x :: 16:32 ____________________
7. x:1 :: 11:1.5 ____________________
8. 50:3 :: 75:x ____________________
9. 67:100 :: 87:x ____________________
10. 78:x :: 100:1 ____________________

Objective

7.5 Solve practical problems using proportions.

Proportions may be used to help solve many types of problems, including drug calculations. Consider the following examples.

Case # 1

You are asked to administer 65 milligrams of intravenous Lidocaine. You know that Lidocaine is packaged 100 mg. in a 5 milliliter prefilled syringe. How many milliliters of Lidocaine will you administer?

Set up your equation as follows by using the known factors. When using unlike terms like milligrams and milliliters, place like terms in places A and C and places B and D as illustrated here.

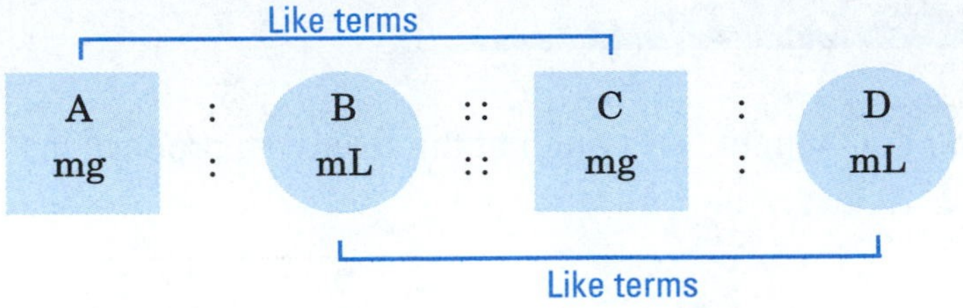

Set up as:

65 mg : x mL :: 100 mg : 5 mL

Find the product of the means and the extremes.

Multiply the means: 65 mg : x mL :: 100 mg : 5 mL

$100 \times x = 100x$

Multiply the extremes: 65 mg : x mL :: 100 mg : 5 mL

$65 \times 5 = 325$

Set up as:

$100x = 325$

To solve for x, divide each side by 100.

$100x \div 100 = 1x$ or x

$325 \div 100 = 3.25$

Solution: $x = 3.25$

Therefore, give 3.25 mL from the syringe to deliver 65 mg of Lidocaine.

Case # 2

Your gross pay is $1,800 and you paid $137.70 to FICA. What percentage of your gross pay is paid to FICA?

Since you know that $1,800 is 100% of your net pay, use 100 to compare against.

The problem:

137.70 : x :: 1,800 : 100

Find the product of the means and the extremes.

Multiply the means: 137.70 : x :: 1,800 : 100

$1{,}800 \times x = 1{,}800x$

Multiply the extremes: 137.70 : x : : 1,800 : 100

137.70 × 100 = 13,770

Set up as:

1,800x = 13,770

To solve for x, divide each side by 1,800.

1,800x ÷ 1,800 = 1x or x

13,770 ÷ 1,800 = 7.65

Solution: x = 7.65

Therefore, your FICA is 7.65% of your gross pay.

SKILL SHARPENER

Solve the following problems.

1. You are asked to administer 30 mg of a medication that is supplied in a 10 mL vial containing 100 mg. How many mL will you give to administer the ordered dose?

   ____

2. The physician orders 500 mg of amoxicillin for an adult patient. Amoxicillin is supplied in 125 mg tablets. How many tablets do you administer?

   ____

3. Acetaminophen is packaged in tablets of 325 mg. The physician asks you to give the resident 650 mg. How many tablets do you give?

   ____

4. You need to administer 4 mg of morphine sulfate (MS) slow IV push. MS is packaged 15 mg per mL. How many milliliters do you administer?

   ____

5. The ratio strength of a solution is 1:10. If there are 10 milliliters of the drug, how many milliliters of the solution are there?

   ____

6. While driving to work last week, you filled the tank of your new car with gasoline. The tank holds 16 gallons. You stopped today and topped off the tank by pumping 9.8 gallons. What percentage of the tank's capacity was left before you refilled the tank today?

   ____

7. Your hourly wage is $14. You are given the opportunity to work on Christmas Day at a rate of $2\frac{1}{2}$ times your normal hourly wage. How much will your hourly wage be if you work on Christmas Day?

____

8. Your patient's urinary output for the shift was 120 mL. What percentage of her total urinary output (of 1,050 mL) for the day occurred on your shift?

____

9. Your company contributes to your retirement fund based on a percentage of your income. You see that the company has contributed $150 to your retirement fund this month. What percentage of your $3,800 salary did your company contribute?

____

10. You can purchase a gross (12 dozen) of 1-inch tape at 83 cents per roll. Individual rolls of the same tape are $1.02 each. Describe the amount (in percent) that you will save if you take advantage of buying tape in bulk.

____

CONCLUSION

Knowing how to use ratios will help you to compare unlike items, and understanding how to solve for missing components in proportions will help you solve everyday problems encountered as a health care provider.

REVIEW AND REFLECT

1. How can you determine if proportions are equal?

____

____

____

____

____

2. Define the term *extremes* as it applies to proportions.

3. Define the term *means* as it applies to proportions.

4. Cite an example of how ratios are used.

5. What mathematical skills are required to solve problems using proportions?

CHAPTER 8

Percentages

LEARNING **OBJECTIVES**

After completing this chapter, the reader will be able to:

- **8.1** Define percent.
- **8.2** Convert decimals to percentages.
- **8.3** Convert percentages to decimals.
- **8.4** Solve to find a percent using multiplication and division.
- **8.5** Solve to find a percent using proportions.

KEY **TERM**

- percent

MATH IN THE REAL WORLD

"Intravenous solutions can be written as decimals or percentages. If the order is written in a decimal, but the solution comes as a percent (and vice versa), then this must be converted to administer the correct solution."

Joyce Mitchell, RN, MSN, MBA

SELF-ASSESSMENT **PRETEST**

Convert the following decimals to percentages.

1. 0.45 ________________

2. 0.78 ________________

3. 0.89 ________________

4. 0.91 ________________

5. 0.3341 ________________

6. 0.2556 ________________

7. 0.873 ________________

8. 0.112 ________________

9. 0.494 ________________

10. 1.00 ________________

Convert the following percentages to decimals.

11. 34% ________________

12. 57% ________________

13. 12% ________________

14. 90% ________________

15. 43% ________________

16. 75.67% ________________

17. 39.44% ________________

18. 11.901% ________________

19. 85.554% ________________

20. 22.450% ________________

Answer the following percentage problems.

21. What is 75% of 350? ________________

22. What is 25.5% of 79? ________________

23. What is 99% of 1,200? ________________

24. What is 23.98% of 125? ________________

25. What is 78.9% of 13,323? ________________

26. What is 1.2% of 5? ________________

27. What is 9.9% of 34? ________________

28. What is 14.95% of 78,000? ________________

29. What is 67% of 32? ______

30. What is 30% of 9? ______

31. 35.1 is what percentage of 78? ______

32. 9.75 is what percentage of 39? ______

33. 111.28 is what percentage of 856? ______

34. 705 is what percentage of 965.8? ______

35. 5.32 is what percentage of 38? ______

36. 56 is what percentage of 175? ______

37. 0.45 is what percentage of 15? ______

38. 47.4 is what percentage of 395? ______

39. 4.5 is what percentage of 250? ______

40. 124.56 is what percentage of 1,384? ______

41. You purchase a television set for $599 and must pay the 9% sales tax. What is your total cost? ______

42. You receive a 7% discount on a purchase of $1,275. What is your discounted cost? ______

43. Your patient's pulse rate is 30% higher than its normal rate of 80. What is her pulse rate? ______

44. All the supplies in the emergency clinic are charged at cost plus 20%. What price would you charge for an item costing $14.75? ______

45. The local fitness club offers memberships for $40 per month. Hospital employees are eligible for a 25% discount. What is the discounted monthly rate for hospital employees? ______

46. Your patient's IV bag holds 1000 mL of normal saline. You see that 350 mL is left. What percentage of the saline has been infused? ______

47. A baseball player reaches base 186 times in 350 at bats. What percentage of the time does he reach base? Round to the nearest hundredth. ______

48. Your passbook savings account pays 3.75% interest on your $3,575 balance. How much interest have you earned? ______

49. How much sales tax would you pay on a purchase of $3.50 based upon a sales tax rate of 8.75%? ______

50. Your hospital reports that 555 of the hospital's 1,500 employees will be eligible for retirement next year. What percentage of the hospital's employees will be eligible for retirement? ______

INTRODUCTION

Health care professionals use percentages in both their daily and professional lives for anything from figuring sale prices, sales tax, and tips to selecting appropriate intravenous solutions, medications, and assessing laboratory values (Figure 8-1). Percentages allow us to easily make comparisons and note changes based on a standard of 100.

Objective

8.1 Define percent.

A **percent** is a part of one hundred. For example, 50% is 50 parts of 100. Though you could write this in other ways, using percentages sometimes makes it easier to understand. Health care providers utilize percentages for figuring discounts, strengths of solutions, and relative changes in anything from oxygen saturation to coronary artery blockage.

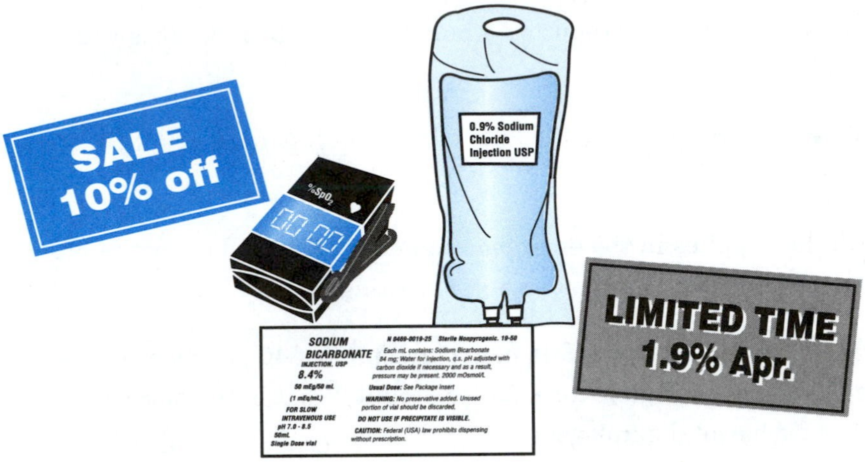

FIGURE 8-1 Whether you realize it or not, we use percentages on a daily basis.

Objective

8.2 Convert decimals to percentages.

To convert decimals to percentages, move the decimal two places to the right and add the % sign to the end. For example, 0.385 becomes 38.5% and 1.7625 becomes 176.25%.

SKILL SHARPENER

Convert the following decimals to percents.

1. 0.375 ______________________
2. 0.0932 ______________________
3. 1.832 ______________________
4. 0.9083 ______________________
5. 2.3323 ______________________
6. 0.3334 ______________________
7. 45.43243 ______________________
8. 1.232 ______________________
9. 0.9823 ______________________
10. 0.6676 ______________________

Objective

8.3 Convert percentages to decimals.

To convert percentages to decimals, remove the % sign and move the decimal two places to the left. For example, 59% would become 0.59.

SKILL SHARPENER

Convert the following percentages to decimals.

1. 34% ______________________
2. 345% ______________________
3. 3.90% ______________________
4. 12.232% ______________________
5. 75.532% ______________________
6. 99.032% ______________________
7. 31.2594% ______________________
8. 54.433% ______________________
9. 8.45% ______________________
10. 92.322% ______________________

Objective

8.4 Solve to find a percent using multiplication and division.

To find a given percent of a number, convert the percentage to a decimal and multiply by the number.

The problem:

Find 63% of 94.

Convert percent to decimal.

$63\% = 0.63$

Multiply.

0.63×94

$$\begin{array}{r} 94 \\ \underline{\times .63} \\ 282 \\ \underline{564} \\ 59.22 \end{array}$$

Solution: 63% of 94 is 59.22

If using a calculator, use the % key.

The problem:

Find 24% of 75.

Push the following buttons to calculate:

[7] [5]

[×]

[2] [4]

[%]

Solution: [18]

To find what percentage of one number another number is, simply divide the number that you want to find the percentage of into the other number. Convert the answer to a percentage.

The problem:

What % of 40 is 8?

Set up as:

$8 \div 40 =$ ______

Divide.

$$\begin{array}{r} .2 \\ 40\overline{)8.0} \\ \underline{8\,0} \\ 0\,0 \end{array}$$

Convert to %.

$$0.2 \times 100 = 20\%$$

Solution: 8 is 20% of 40.

SKILL SHARPENER

Answer the following questions.

1. What is 75% of 350? __________
2. What is 40% of $12.95? __________
3. What is 99% of 250? __________
4. What is 12% of 32? __________
5. What is 25% of 3,200? __________
6. What is 19% of 15? __________
7. What is 5% of 150? __________
8. What is 34% of 88? __________
9. What is 65% of 65? __________
10. What is 8% of 185? __________
11. What percentage of 12 is 4? __________
12. What percentage of 900 is 180? __________
13. What percentage of 750 is 50? __________
14. What percentage of 120 is 100? __________
15. What percentage of 300 is 75? __________
16. What percentage of 250 is 75? __________
17. What percentage of 76 is 14? __________
18. What percentage of 88 is 3? __________
19. What percentage of 12.5 is 8? __________
20. What percentage of 3.5 is 1.25? __________

Objective

8.5 Solve to find a percent using proportions.

Another way to find a percent is by using proportions. Set up your proportion by using **x** to indicate the unknown factor and **100** to signify 100%.

The problem:

What % of 150 is 120?

Note: Since we are finding a percentage (part of 100) we will use 100 as the whole.

Because 150 is the other whole, set up the equation as:

x : 100 :: 120 : 150

Multiply the means: x : 100 :: 120 : 150

$100 \times 120 = 12{,}000$

Multiply the extremes: x : 100 :: 120 : 150

$150 \times x = 150x$

Set up as:

$12{,}000 = 150x$

To solve for x, divide each side by 150.

$12{,}000 \div 150 = 80$

$150x \div 150 = 1x$ or x

Solution: x = 80

Therefore, 80 : 100 :: 120 : 150 or 120 is 80% of 150.

By utilizing proportions, you can determine the missing component regardless which component is missing.

SKILL SHARPENER

Solve the following word problems using proportions.

1. What is 34% of 325? ____________________

2. What is 75% of 150? ____________________

3. What is 12.5% of 325? ____________________

4. What is 34.58% of 76? ______________________

5. What is 1.9% of 768? ______________________

6. What is 5.47% of 9,380? ______________________

7. What is 3.75% of 36? ______________________

8. What is 7% of 99? ______________________

9. What is 33.35% of 190? ______________________

10. What is 5.8% of 346? ______________________

11. What percentage of 150 is 18.75? ______________________

12. What percentage of 398 is 294.52? ______________________

13. What percentage of 125 is 27.5? ______________________

14. What percentage of 1,395 is 153.45? ______________________

15. What percentage of 69 is 35.88? ______________________

16. What percentage of 12 is 4.32? ______________________

17. What percentage of 1,965 is 137.55? ______________________

18. What percentage of 550 is 247.5? ______________________

19. What percentage of 475 is 460.75? ______________________

20. What percentage of 1,200 is 30.72? ______________________

CONCLUSION

Percentages are used in many ways, in both health care and daily life, to make numbers and relationships between numbers easier to understand. The ability to convert from decimals to percentages and percentages to decimals, along with the ability to find a percentage using multiplication, division, and proportions, will be beneficial in both your professional career and your personal life.

REVIEW AND REFLECT

1. In what ways are percents used in everyday life?

2. How does using a percent make it easier to compare figures?

3. Describe what percent means.

4. If 100% represents all of something, why do we sometimes have more than 100%?

5. Determine what percentage of your time is spent sleeping, at school, watching television, and studying. One hour is equal to what percent of a day?

CHAPTER 9

Conversions

LEARNING OBJECTIVES

After completing this chapter, the reader will be able to:

- **9.1** Convert from decimal to fraction.
- **9.2** Convert from decimal to percent.
- **9.3** Convert from fraction to decimal.
- **9.4** Convert from fraction to percent.
- **9.5** Convert from percent to fraction.
- **9.6** Convert from percent to decimal.
- **9.7** Convert units of measure within the metric system.
- **9.8** Convert units of measure within the apothecary system.
- **9.9** Convert units of measure within the household system.
- **9.10** Convert between the apothecary, household, and metric systems.

KEY TERM

- conversion

MATH IN THE REAL WORLD

"An order may read to give 250 mg of Rocephin (injectable antibiotic), but the computer will only let us record the medication in grams, so I need to record it as 0.25 grams in the computer."

Joyce Mitchell, RN, MSN, MBA

SELF-ASSESSMENT **PRETEST**

Convert the following to fractions.

1. 0.44 ______

2. 0.68 ______

3. 0.23 ______

4. 0.11 ______

5. 0.98 ______

6. 0.77 ______

7. 0.875 ______

8. 0.34 ______

9. 0.125 ______

10. 0.900 ______

Convert the following to percents.

11. 0.46 ______

12. 0.125 ______

13. 0.33 ______

14. 0.87 ______

15. 0.58 ______

16. 0.91 ______

17. 0.74 ______

18. 0.24 ______

19. 0.650 ______

20. 0.312 ______

Convert the following to decimals.

21. $\frac{4}{9}$ ______

22. $\frac{9}{10}$ ______

23. $\frac{34}{50}$ ____________________

24. $\frac{22}{40}$ ____________________

25. $\frac{12}{15}$ ____________________

26. $\frac{7}{16}$ ____________________

27. $\frac{3}{9}$ ____________________

28. $\frac{55}{65}$ ____________________

29. $\frac{9}{11}$ ____________________

30. $\frac{51}{75}$ ____________________

Convert the following to percents.

31. $\frac{41}{55}$ ____________________

32. $\frac{3}{8}$ ____________________

33. $\frac{6}{90}$ ____________________

34. $\frac{2}{3}$ ____________________

35. $\frac{4}{11}$ ____________________

36. $\frac{9}{20}$ ____________________

37. $\frac{64}{66}$ ____________________

38. $\frac{21}{30}$ ____________________

39. $\frac{7}{19}$ ____________________

40. $\frac{23}{35}$ ____________________

Convert the following to fractions.

41. 34% ____________________

42. 57% ____________________

43. 87% ____________________

44. 66% ____________________

45. 12% ____________________

46. 12.5% ____________________

47. 77% ____________________

48. 80% ____________________

49. 42.9% ____________________

50. 23% ____________________

Convert the following to decimals.

51. 13% ____________________

52. 61% ____________________

53. 59% ____________________

54. 31% ____________________

55. 98% ____________________

56. 50% ____________________

57. 66% ____________________

58. 80% ____________________

59. 34% ____________________

60. 99% ____________________

Convert the following measurements.

61. 3 g = ______ kg

62. 12 km = ______ m

63. 1300 mg = ______ g

64. 0.595 l = ______ mL

65. 4 dr = ______ gr

66. 16 fl ʒ = ______ fl ℥

67. 4 pt = ______ qt

68. 540 drops = ______ T

69. 2 glasses = ______ fluidounces

70. 4 T = ______ t

INTRODUCTION

One of the most important mathematical skills health care providers need is the ability to convert from one unit of measurement to another. **Conversion** is the act of changing from one system or measurement to another. Sometimes this skill involves conversion from a decimal to a percent. Sometimes it involves conversions to or from fractions. It may involve conversion between measurement systems. This chapter helps you practice converting from one type of number to another and one type of measurement system to another.

Objective

9.1 Convert from decimal to fraction.

Sometimes you will need to convert from a decimal to a fraction. To do this, follow the steps outlined below.

The problem:

Convert 0.84 to a fraction.

Since we know that 0.84 is equal to $\frac{84}{100}$, we can convert to $\frac{84}{100}$ and reduce.

To reduce, find the greatest common factor (GCF) of the numerator and denominator.

84	100
$1 \times 84 = 84$	$1 \times 100 = 100$
$2 \times 42 = 84$	$2 \times 50 = 100$
$4 \times 21 = 84$	$4 \times 25 = 100$

The GCF is 4.

Divide the numerator and denominator by the GCF.

$$\frac{84 \div 4}{100 \div 4} = \frac{21}{25}$$

Solution: $0.84 = \frac{21}{25}$

SKILL SHARPENER

Convert the following decimals to fractions. Reduce to lowest terms.

1. 0.38 ____________________

2. 0.97 ____________________

3. 0.233 ________________

4. 0.125 ________________

5. 0.25 ________________

6. 0.75 ________________

7. 0.9 ________________

8. 1.23 ________________

9. 2.75 ________________

10. 3.5 ________________

Objective

9.2 Convert from decimal to percent.

To convert from a decimal to a percent, move the decimal two places to the right and add a % sign. For example, 0.50 equals 50%.

SKILL SHARPENER

Convert the following decimals to percents.

1. 0.34 ________________

2. 0.25 ________________

3. 0.87 ________________

4. 0.67 ________________

5. 0.39 ________________

6. 0.2 ________________

7. 0.9 ____________________

8. 0.123 ____________________

9. 1.23 ____________________

10. 2.78 ____________________

Objective

9.3 Convert from fraction to decimal.

To convert a fraction to a decimal, divide the denominator into the numerator. The quotient is your answer.

The problem:

Convert $\frac{3}{5}$ to a decimal.

Set up as:

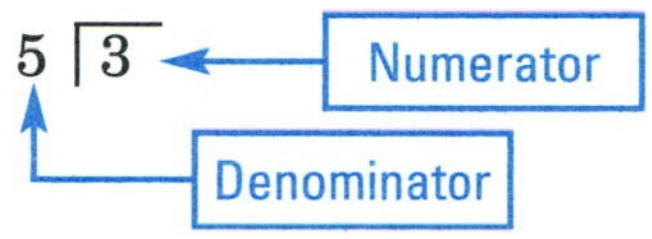

Divide.

$$\begin{array}{r} 0.6 \\ 5\,\overline{)\,3.0} \\ \underline{3\,0} \\ 0 \end{array}$$

Solution: $\frac{3}{5} = 0.6$

If the dividend repeats the same digit, place a line over the repeating digits or use rounding to complete your answer. Consider this example.

The problem:

Convert $\frac{1}{3}$ to a decimal.

Set up as:

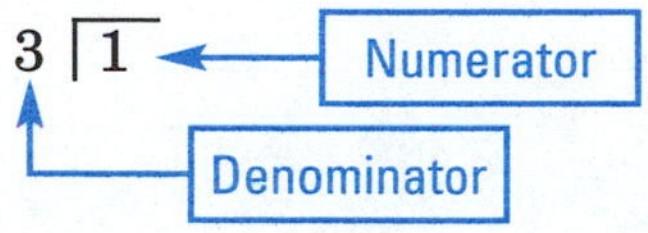

Divide.

$$\begin{array}{r} 0.333 \\ 3\,\overline{)\,1.000} \\ \underline{9} \\ 10 \\ \underline{9} \\ 10 \end{array}$$

Solution: $\frac{1}{3} = 0.\overline{33}$

Since the 3 will keep repeating indefinitely, place a line over the 3s.

SKILL SHARPENER

Convert the following fractions to decimals.

1. $\frac{1}{2}$ ____________________

2. $\frac{2}{3}$ ____________________

3. $\frac{4}{5}$ ____________________

4. $\frac{7}{16}$ ____________________

5. $\frac{9}{10}$ ____________________

6. $\frac{32}{100}$ ____________________

7. $\frac{3}{8}$ ____________________

8. $\frac{8}{16}$ ____________________

9. $\frac{3}{9}$ ____________________

10. $\frac{125}{1000}$ ____________________

Objective

9.4 Convert from fraction to percent.

To convert from a fraction to a percent, first convert the fraction to a decimal. To accomplish this, divide the denominator into the numerator.

The problem:

Convert $\frac{3}{8}$ to a percent.

Set up as:

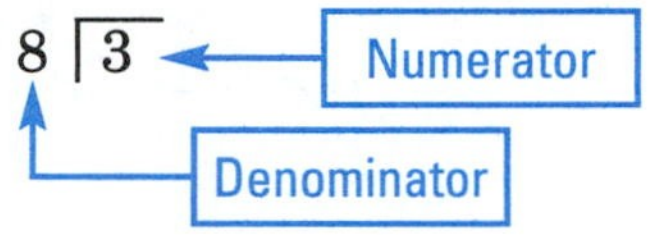

Divide.

```
    0.375
8 | 3.000
    24
     60
     56
      40
```

Convert decimal to percent by moving the decimal two spaces to the right and add the % sign.

0.37.5

Solution: $\frac{3}{8} = 37.5\%$

SKILL SHARPENER

Convert the following fractions to percents.

1. $\frac{4}{5}$ ____________________

2. $\frac{2}{3}$ ____________________

3. $\frac{1}{8}$ ____________________

4. $\frac{6}{7}$ ____________________

5. $\frac{3}{9}$ ______________________

6. $\frac{12}{36}$ ______________________

7. $\frac{23}{45}$ ______________________

8. $\frac{45}{150}$ ______________________

9. $\frac{7}{16}$ ______________________

10. $\frac{8}{32}$ ______________________

Objective

9.5 Convert from percent to fraction.

To convert from a percent to a fraction, first convert the percent to a decimal. That decimal number should be used as the numerator and the denominator should be 100. Then reduce to the lowest terms.

The problem:

Convert 37% to a fraction.

Convert to a decimal by dropping the % sign and moving the decimal two places to the left.

37%

0.37. — Drop % and move decimal two places to the left.

0.37

Since we know that 0.37 is equal to $\frac{37}{100}$, we should now reduce to lowest terms.

To reduce, find the GCF of the numerator and denominator.

37	100
1 × 37 = 37	1 × 100 = 100
	2 × 50 = 100
	4 × 25 = 100
	5 × 20 = 100
	10 × 10 = 100

Since the GCF is 1, this cannot be reduced any further.

Solution: $37\% = \frac{37}{100}$

SKILL SHARPENER

Convert the following percents to fractions. Reduce to lowest terms.

1. 23% ________________

2. 45% ________________

3. 90% ________________

4. 50% ________________

5. 33% ________________

6. 65% ________________

7. 60% ________________

8. 12% ________________

9. 9% ________________

10. 125% ________________

Objective

9.6 Convert from percent to decimal.

When converting from a percent to a decimal, simply drop the % sign and move the decimal two places to the left.

The problem:

Convert 98% to a decimal.

Drop the % sign and move the decimal two places to the left.

98%

0.98.

0.98

Solution: 98% = 0.98

SKILL SHARPENER

Convert the following percents to decimals.

1. 32% __________

2. 15% __________

3. 67% __________

4. 324% __________

5. 3% __________

6. 13% __________

7. 91% __________

8. 0.38% ____________________

9. 0.9% ____________________

10. 12% ____________________

Objective

9.7 Convert units of measure within the metric system.

Since the metric system is based on units of ten, conversion requires that you multiply or divide. This is made especially simple since multiplication and division may be accomplished by moving decimals to the right or left.

To multiply by 10, move the decimal one place to the right.

Example

39.84 × 10 =

39.84

398.4

To multiply by 100 — move the decimal 2 places to the right.
To multiply by 1,000 — move the decimal 3 places to the right.
To multiply by 10,000 — move the decimal 4 places to the right.
To multiply by 100,000 — move the decimal 5 places to the right.

To divide by 10, move the decimal one place to the left.

Example

39.84 ÷ 10 =

39.84

3.984

To divide by 100 — move the decimal 2 places to the left.
To divide by 1,000 — move the decimal 3 places to the left.
To divide by 10,000 — move the decimal 4 places to the left.
To divide by 100,000 — move the decimal 5 places to the left.

SKILL SHARPENER

Convert the following measurements.

1. 56 g = ________ kg

2. 260 mL = ________ L

3. 3.4 L = ________ hL

4. 24 km = ________ m

5. 2,300 cm = ________ dm

6. 0.5 L = ________ mL

7. 29 mg = ________ g

8. 3,400 mg = ________ g

9. 2.3 L = ________ mL

10. 0.125 L = ________ mL

Objective

9.8 Convert units of measure within the apothecary system.

To convert units of measure within the apothecary system, refer to the conversion chart shown in Figure 9-1.

60 grains (gr)	=	1 dram (dr) ʒ
8 drams (dr)	=	1 ounce (oz) ℥
12 ounces (oz)	=	1 pound (lb)
60 minims (♏)	=	1 fluidram (fldr)
8 fluidrams (fldr)	=	1 fluidounce (floz)
16 fluidounces (floz)	=	1 pint (pt)
2 pints (pt)	=	1 quart (qt)
4 quarts (qt)	=	1 gallon (gal)

FIGURE 9-1 Apothecary equivalents

Conversions may easily be made by using proportions. Consider this example.

The problem:

> The medication order reads ʒss. You need to figure how many grains to administer.

Since we know that 1 dram is equivalent to 60 grains, set up the problem as a proportion.

Set up as:

$$\frac{1}{2} \text{ dram} : x \text{ grains} :: 1 \text{ dram} : 60 \text{ grains}$$

Multiply the means. $\frac{1}{2} : x :: 1 : 60$

$$1 \times x = 1x \text{ or } x$$

Multiply the extremes. $\frac{1}{2} : x :: 1 : 60$

$$\frac{1}{2} \times 60 = 30$$

Solution: x = 30

Therefore, $\frac{1}{2}$ dram = 30 grains.

SKILL SHARPENER

Convert the following measurements.

1. 60 gr = ________ dr
2. 2 dr = ________ gr
3. 16 floz = ________ pt
4. 2 pt = ________ qt
5. 4 fldr = ________ ♍
6. 8 fldr = ________ floz
7. 2 gal = ________ qt

8. 1 gal = ________ pt

9. 480 ♏ = ________ floz

10. 1 fldr = ________ ♏

Objective

9.9 Convert units of measure within the household system.

To convert units of measure within the household system, refer to the conversion chart in Figure 9-2.

60 gtt	=	1 t or tsp		
3 t or tsp	=	1 T		
180 gtt	=	1 T	=	$\frac{1}{2}$ oz
2 T	=	1 oz	=	6 t or tsp
360 gtt	=	2 T		
1 oz	=	30 cc or 30 mL		
6 oz	=	1 tcp		
8 oz	=	1 C or 1 glass		
2 C	=	1 pt	=	16 oz
2 pt	=	1 qt	=	32 oz
4 C	=	1 qt	=	32 oz
4 qt	=	1 gal	=	128 oz

FIGURE 9-2 Household equivalents

Make conversions using proportions as illustrated here.

The problem:

> Your patient needs 30 mL of a liquid medication. You know that 30 mL is equivalent to 1 ounce, and $\frac{1}{2}$ ounce is roughly equivalent to 1 T.

Set up as:

30 mL : x T :: 15 mL : 1 T

Multiply the means. 30 : x :: 15 : 1

$x \times 15 = 15x$

Multiply the extremes. 30 : x :: 15 : 1

$30 \times 1 = 30$

$15x = 30$

To solve for x, divide both sides by 15.

$15x \div 15 = 1x$ or x

$30 \div 15 = 2$

Solution: x = 2

Therefore, 2 T = 30 mL.

SKILL SHARPENER

Convert the following measurements.

1. 60 drops = ________ t

2. 240 drops = ________ T

3. 1 glass = ________ ounces

4. 1 cup = ________ oz

5. 1 oz = ________ T

6. 1 T = ________ t

7. 4 T = ________ oz

8. 1 ounce = ________ drops

9. 12 ounces = ________ cup

10. 3 T = ________ t

Objective

9.10 Convert between the apothecary, household, and metric systems.

Health care providers are frequently asked to convert from one measurement system to another. It is important that care is taken to assure accuracy in conversions. Since proportions may be used to compare unlike items, it is an ideal method to convert between the systems of measurement. Appendix C contains conversion charts for the three common systems of measurement.

The problem:

> You need to instruct a patient how to take 8 drams (ʒ) of a medication. Since you know that one dram is equivalent to 2 teaspoons, convert to a measure that the patient can use at home.

Set up as:

8 drams : x tsp :: 1 dram : 2 tsp

Multiply the means. 8 : x :: 1 : 2

$x \times 1 = 1x$ or x

Multiply the extremes. 8 : x :: 1 : 2

$8 \times 2 = 16$

Solution: x = 16

Therefore, to take 8 drams, the patient must take 16 tsp.

What is another way you could make it easier for the patient to take the medicine? Could you convert to another household measure?

SKILL SHARPENER

Convert the following measurements using proportions.

1. 1 oz = ________ gtts

2. 1 pt = ________ mL

3. 60 mL = ________ drop

4. 1 T = ________ gtts

5. 1 T = ________ mL

6. 4 T = ________ mL

7. 30 ♍ = ________ mL

8. 2 floz = ________ mL

9. 10 mL = ________ fl ʒ

10. 1 floz = ________ T

CONCLUSION

Using the skills in this chapter, you should be able to make necessary conversions between fractions, decimals, and percents. Though it may not be necessary to perform these conversions on a daily basis, the ability to perform these conversions will make your job as a health care professional easier and will help you to provide the best care for your patients.

Your ability to convert between each of the three systems of measurement is important in assuring that patients receive the correct dosages of medications, both while in your care and at home. It is helpful to memorize some of the common conversions and to keep a chart, like the one in Appendix C, handy for those less common conversions.

REVIEW AND REFLECT

1. Describe one situation in which you may need to convert between fractions and decimals.

2. Describe one situation in which you may need to convert between decimals and percents.

3. Why is it important to be able to help patients convert medications from metric and apothecary measurements to household measurements?

4. Explain why you move the decimal two places to the left when converting from a percent to a decimal.

5. Describe another method of converting from fractions to decimals.

UNIT 3

Applications

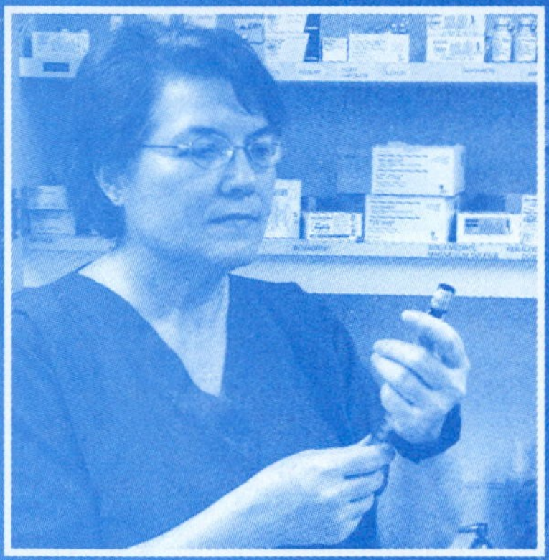

This unit allows the student to apply the skills learned in Unit Two to actual examples that are relevant and mimic those experienced in the work place. Through practice, these operations will become second nature as they develop into part of the health care professional's daily routine.

Though some operations may seem routine, students should realize that accuracy is imperative, and attention to detail is crucial in assuring that patients receive the best possible care.

CHAPTER 10

Medication Dosage Calculations

LEARNING OBJECTIVES

After completing this chapter, the reader will be able to:

- **10.1** List the components of a typical medication label.
- **10.2** Read a medication label.
- **10.3** Read a prescription.
- **10.4** Read a syringe.
- **10.5** Determine the amount of fluid remaining in an intravenous bag.
- **10.6** Calculate intravenous drip rates.
- **10.7** Determine the concentration of solutions.
- **10.8** Calculate medication dosages using proportions.
- **10.9** Convert medication dosages for home use.

KEY TERMS

- concentration of a solution
- drip rate
- expiration date
- generic name
- KVO line
- lot number
- macrodrip
- medication label
- microdrip
- percent strength
- piggyback
- prescription
- syringe
- TKO line
- trade name

MATH IN THE REAL WORLD

"Many medication doses are based on how much the patient weighs. For example, I want to prescribe 20 mg/kg of a drug to a patient. How do I calculate the appropriate total dose when all I have is the weight in pounds? Also, some drugs are dispensed using old apothecary measurements such as grains. What does

that mean in the metric system, which happens to be the mathematical language of scientific measurement?"

Laurie Romig, MD, FACEP

"You only have one opportunity to administer to the patient the correct dosage of medication...no matter how many years you practice, never violate your fundamentals...read the label three times. It is not illegal, immoral, or unethical to have caused a drug error but an attempt to conceal it violates all three."

Mike Harper, CRNA, JD

SELF-ASSESSMENT **PRETEST**

Label the components of this medication label.

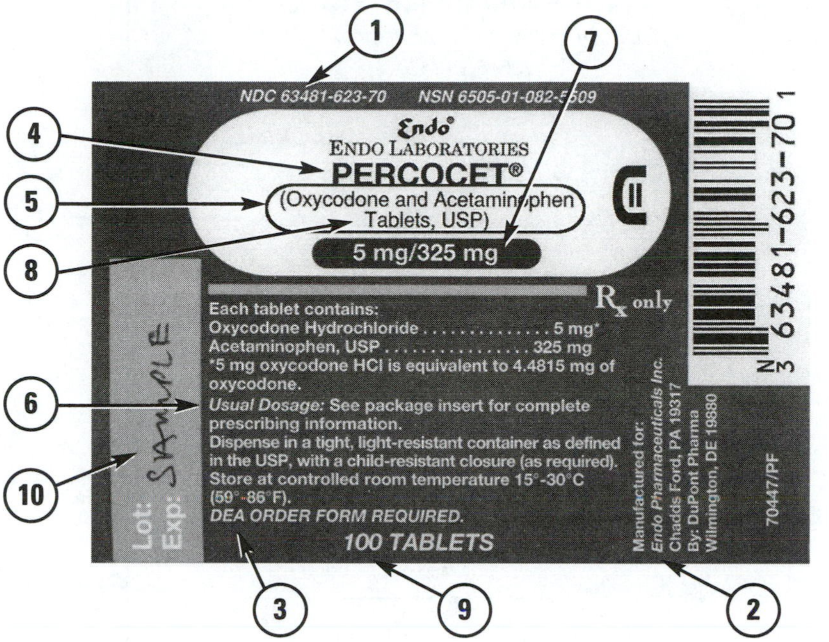

1. ______________________________

2. ______________________________

3. ______________________________

4. ______________________________

5. ______________________________

6. ______________________________

7. ______________________________

8. ______________________________

9. ______________________________

10. ______________________________

Label the components of this prescription.

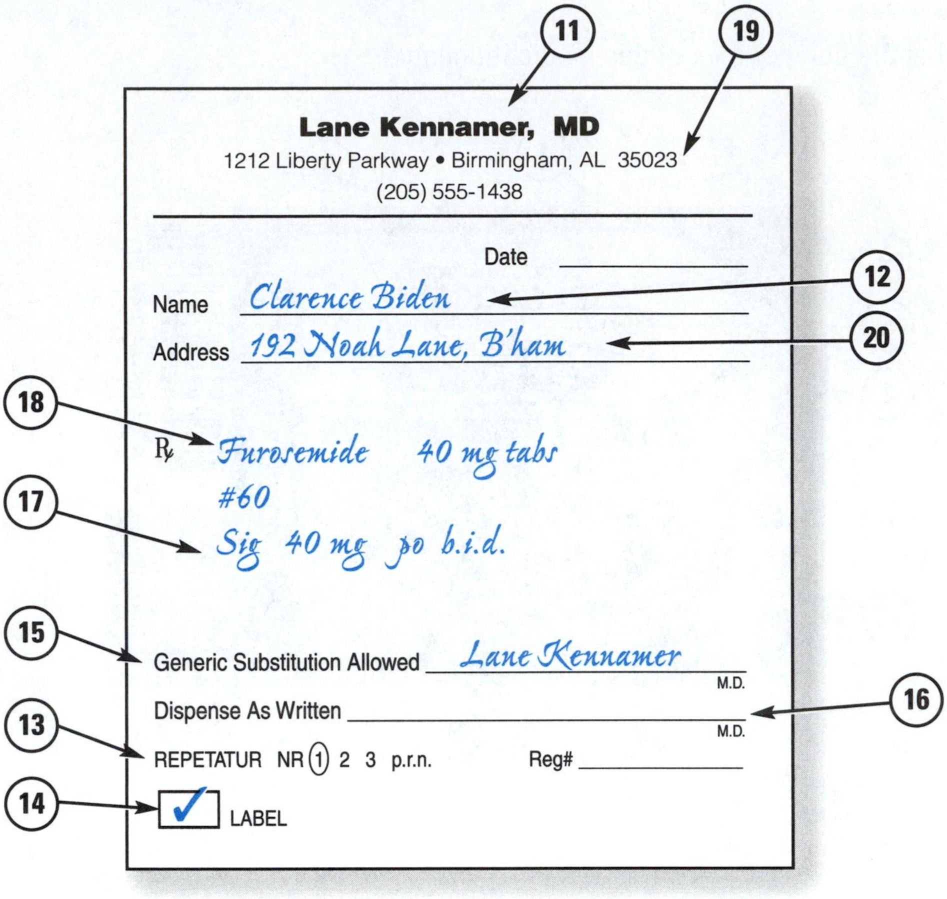

11. ______________________

12. ______________________

13. ______________________

14. ______________________

15. ______________________

16. ______________________

17. ______________________

18. ______________________

19. ______________________

20. ______________________

Determine the amount of solution remaining in each of the following syringes.

21. ______________________________

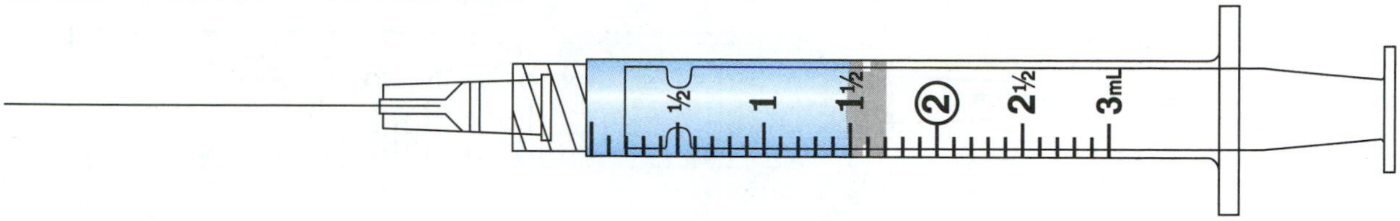

22. ______________________________

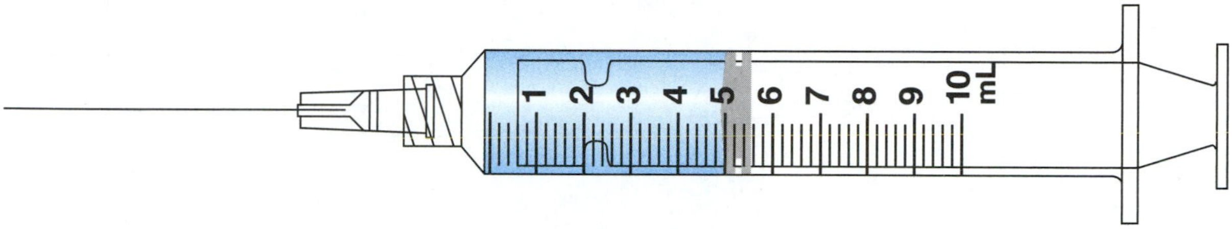

23. ______________________________

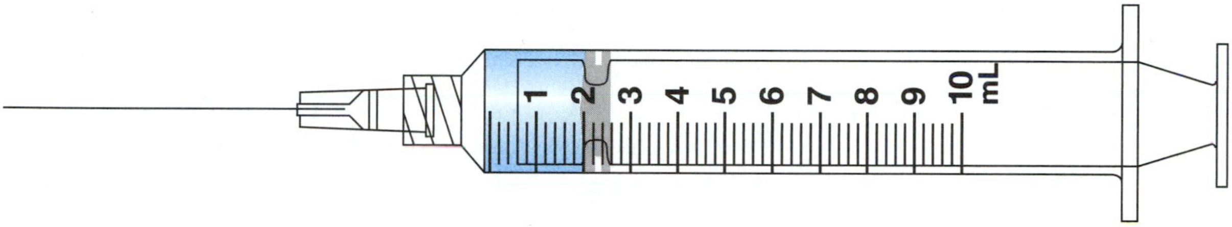

24. ______________________________

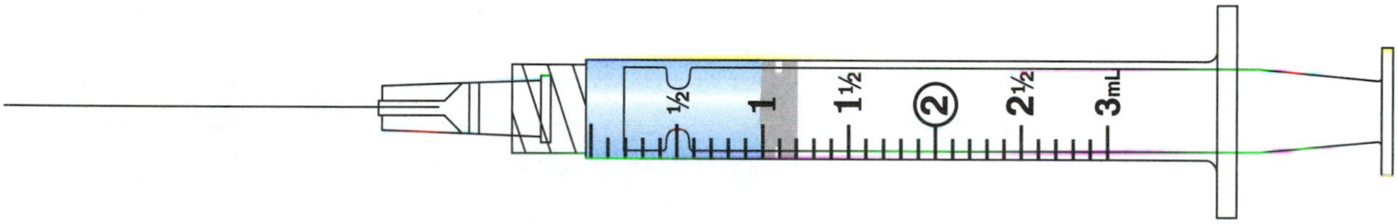

25. ______________________________

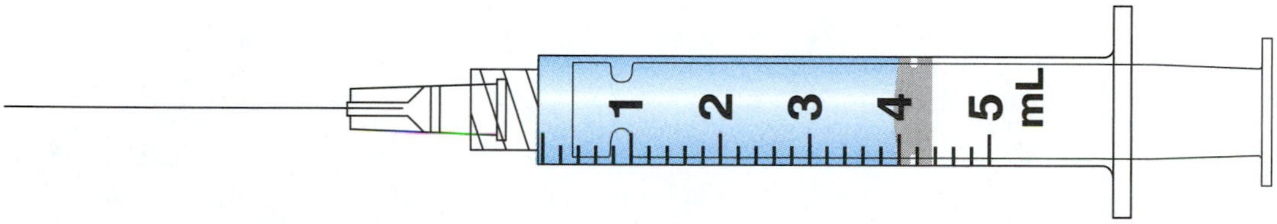

26. ______________________________

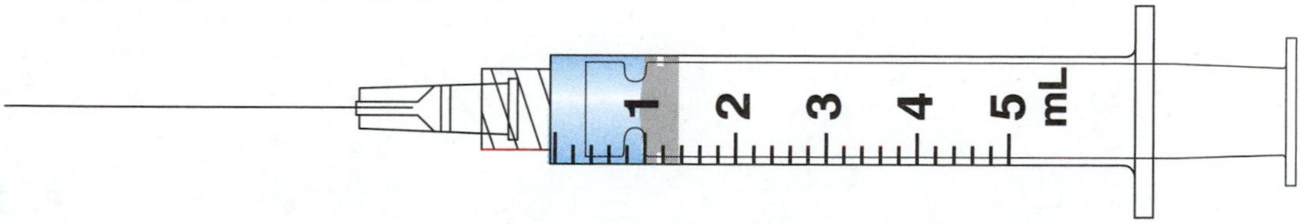

27. ______________________________

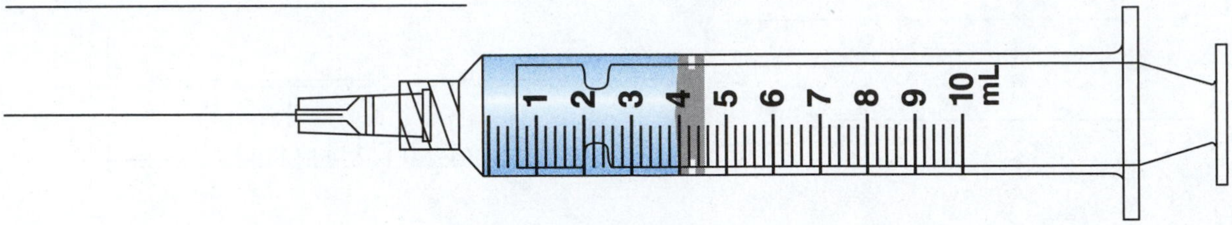

28. ______________________________

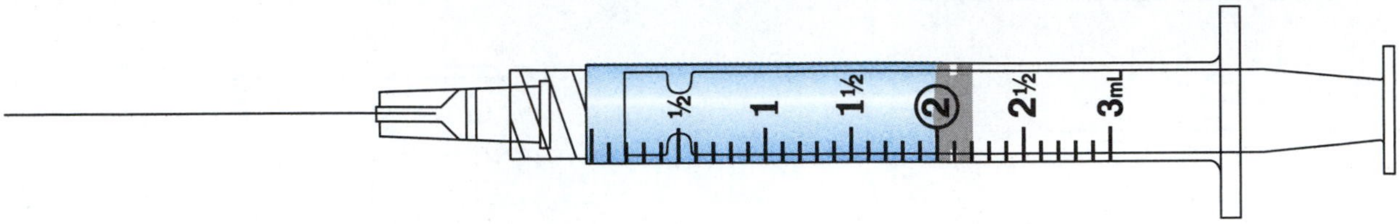

29. ______________________________

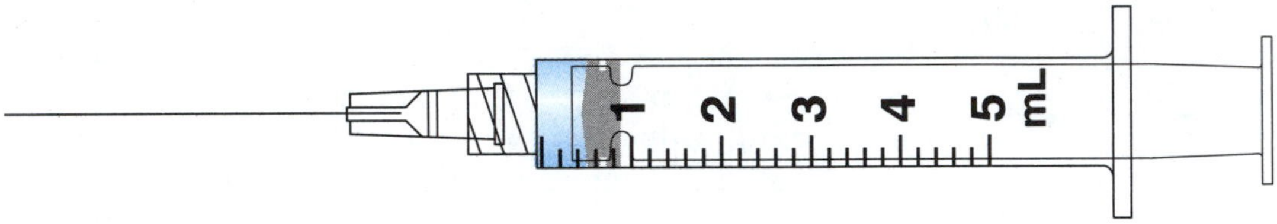

30. ______________________________

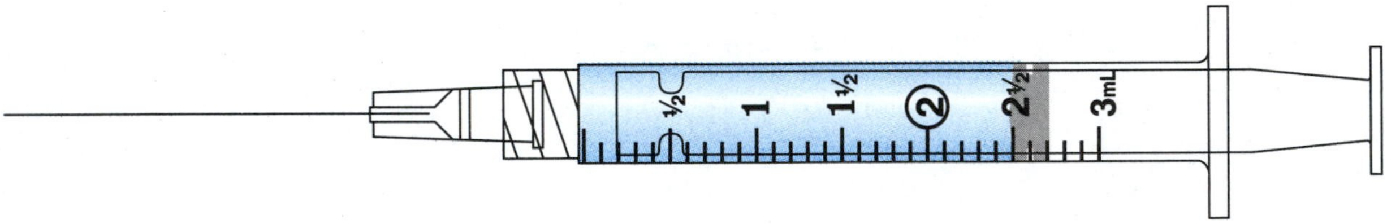

Determine the amount of solution remaining in each of the following IV bags.

31. ______________________________

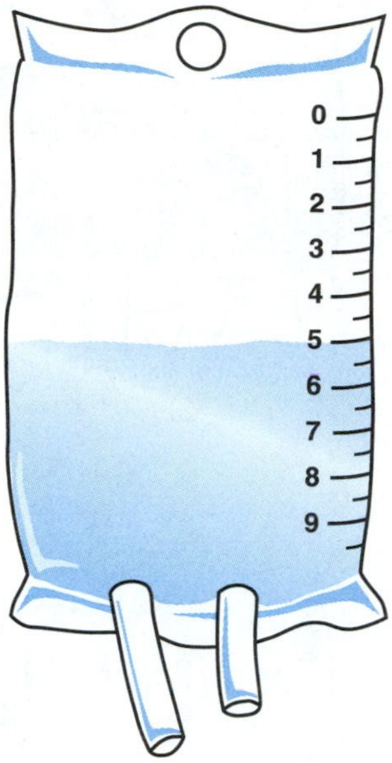

32. ______________________________

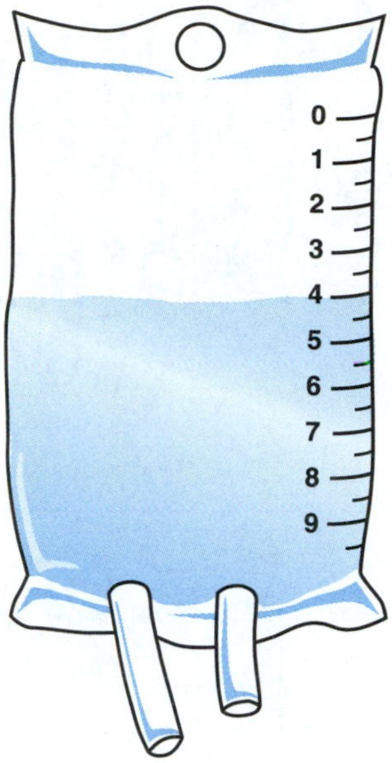

33. ______________________________

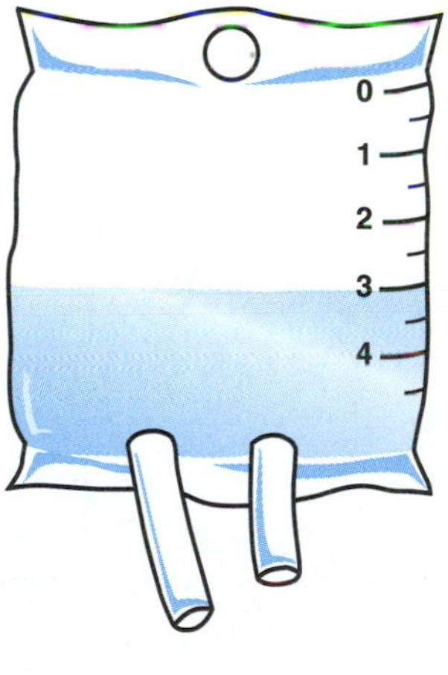

34. ______________________________

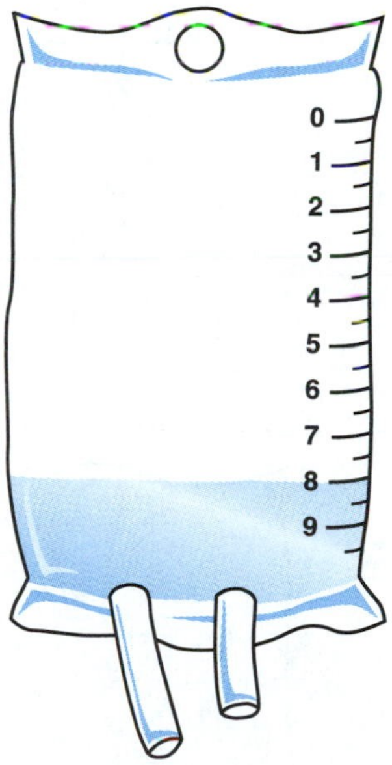

35. ______________________

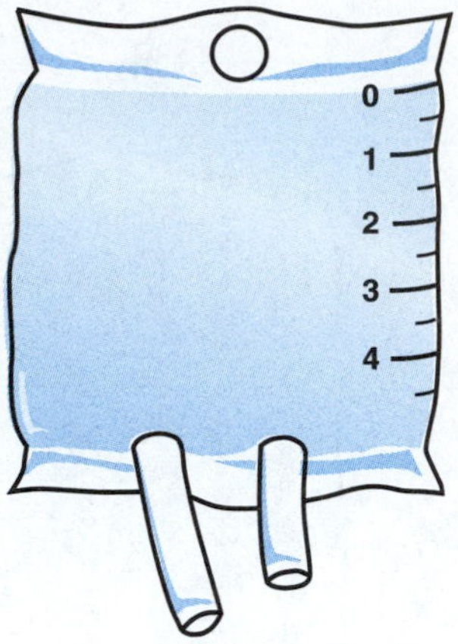

36. ______________________

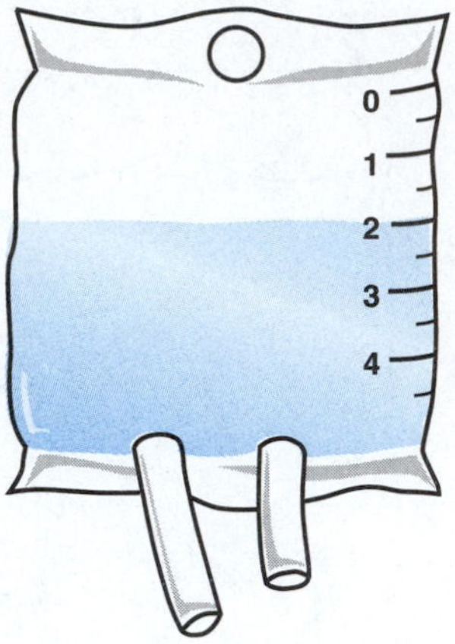

37. ______________________

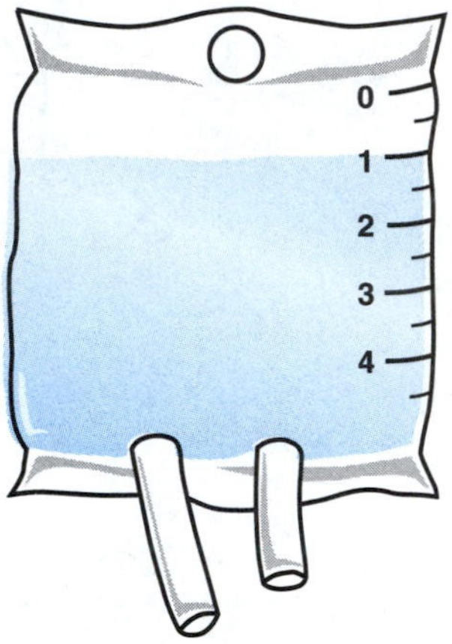

38. ______________________

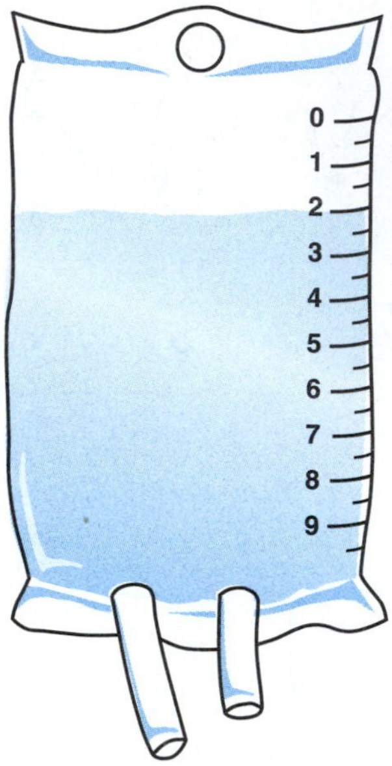

39. ______________________

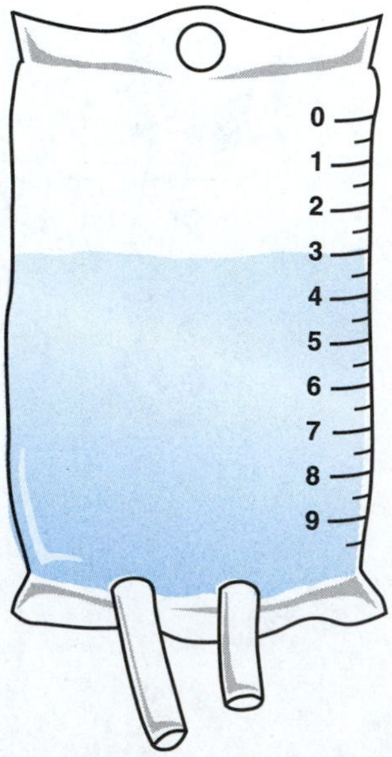

40. ______________________

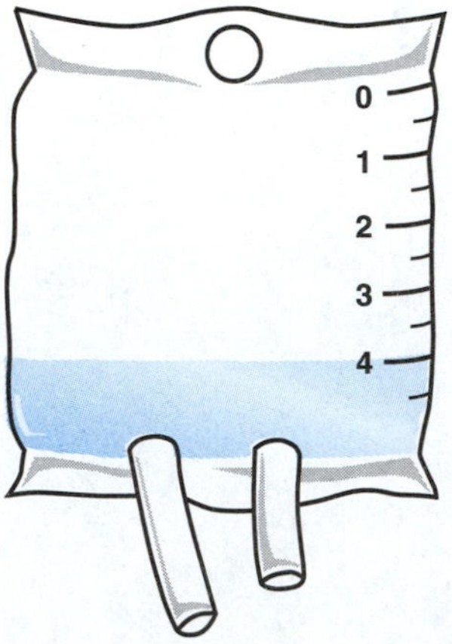

Calculate the following IV drip rates.

41. You need to administer 250 mL of normal saline over a 3-hour period using a 15-drop set. ____________________

42. Administer 125 mL of lactated ringers in 1 hour using a 12-drop set. ____________________

43. Administer 750 mL of saline over 12 hours using a 10-drop set. ____________________

44. You are asked to administer 300 mL of fluid over 90 minutes using a 15-drop set. ____________________

45. You need to administer 400 mL of normal saline over a 2-hour period using a 10-drop set. ____________________

Indicate the solute-to-solvent ratio in the following, first by using a ratio (x:100) and then by converting to a percentage (x%).

46. 8 parts of a mineral in 100 parts of liquid ________ :100 ________ %

47. 12 parts of a drug in 100 parts of water ________ :100 ________ %

48. 25 parts of glucose in 100 parts water ________ :100 ________ %

49. 1.5 parts drug in 10 parts water ________ :100 ________ %

50. 3 parts of a mineral in 100 parts water ________ :100 ________ %

How much of the solvent (drug or mineral) must be given to attain the following solutions? Figure using proportions and show your work.

51. 12 mL of a 3% solution ______________

52. 200 mL of a 2% solution ______________

53. 30 mL of a 9% solution ______________

54. 5 mL of a 4% solution ______________

55. 10 mL of a 0.5% solution ______________

In each of the following, use proportions to determine the volume of medication to be given.

56. You must administer 75 mg of Lidocaine. It is packaged in a prefilled syringe with 100 mg in 5 mL of solution. ______________

57. Epinephrine is packaged 1 mg/mL in a 10 mL vial. How many mL do you administer if you wish to give 3 mg? ______________

58. A drug is packaged 0.5 mg per mL. How many mL do you give if your order is for 3.5 mg? ______________

59. You are asked to give 5 mg of Tenormin. It is supplied 1 mg/2 mL in a 10 mL ampule. ____________________

60. Oxytocin is packaged in a 1 mL ampule that contains 10 units. How many mL do you give when administering 6 units? ____________________

Using the household system of measurement, write in simple terms how much and how often the patient should take the prescribed medicine.

61. Take 1/200 gr SL prn chest pain. Tablets are supplied as 0.3 mg.

____

____

____

62. The physician orders 0.75 g to take PO t.i.d. Capsules come in 250 mg strength.

____

____

____

63. Direct the patient to take 240 mg PO b.i.d. until gone. The prescription says to dispense #42, 80 mg tablets.

____

____

____

64. The physician orders 1 dr of solution b.i.d.

____

____

____

65. Explain to the patient to take 2 dr of elixir PO q.i.d.

____

____

____

INTRODUCTION

Health care providers deal with medication dosages and solution strengths in a number of ways. Your ability to perform mathematical calculations and accurately read medication orders and labels will help assure that patients receive the correct dosages and strengths of the intended medicines. Additionally, it is important that you be able to interpret medication orders and convert medication orders to household measurements so that patients accurately measure their medications using household devices.

Objective

10.1 List the components of a typical medication label.

It is important that health care professionals be able to read a **medication label**. These labels contain important information that helps the health care professional to assure that the right medication at the right strength is delivered to the patient. Though the style of medication labels varies, certain components should be common to each label.

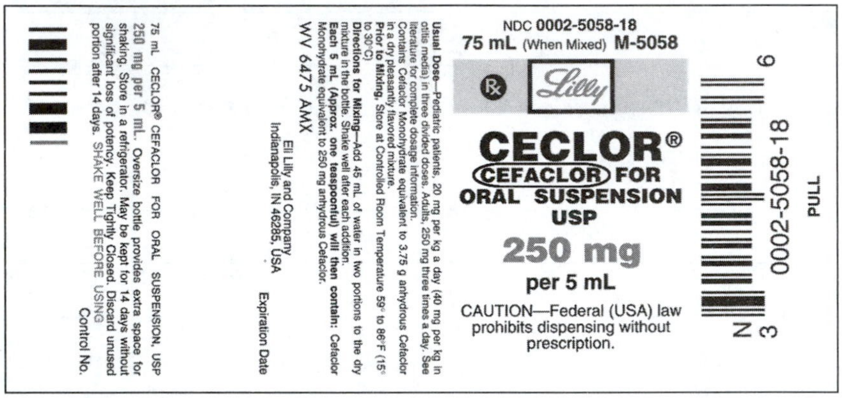

Trade name – Also referred to as brand name of the medication

Generic name – The nonproprietary name of the medication

Manufacturer – The company that manufactured the medication

National Drug Code (NDC) number – A number used to identify the manufacturer, the medication, and the container size

Dosage strength – Amount of medication contained within a given dose (in this example, 250 mg per 5 mL)

Drug form – Whether a liquid, capsule, drop, tablet, and so on

Usual adult dose – The typical adult dose for the common use of the medicine

Total amount enclosed – Number of tablets, approximate number of drops, ounces, or milliliters

Prescription warning – Denotes that this medication is available by prescription only

Expiration date – Denotes the last date in which this medication should be used (Since this label is for purposes of illustration, no expiration date is visible.)

Lot or control number – The lot number would be applied before shipping the actual product (In this example, there is no lot number visible.)

SKILL SHARPENER

Find the requested information on each of the following medication labels or boxes. If you are unable to see one of the requested items, write "NOT SEEN" on the line.

1.

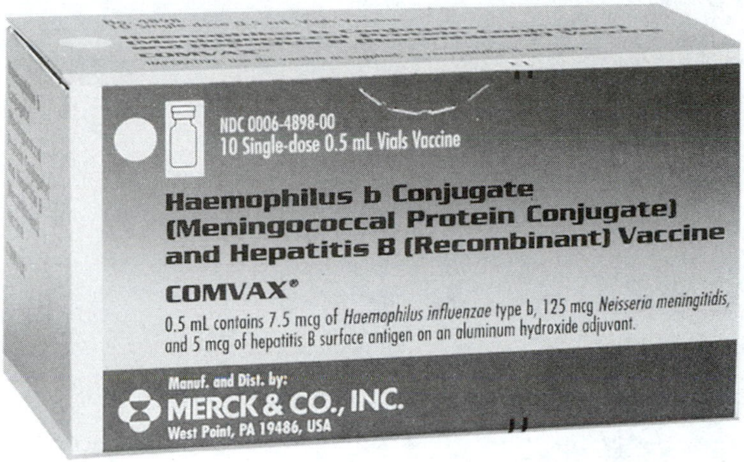

Trade name ____________________

Generic name ____________________

Manufacturer ____________________

NDC number ____________________

Dosage strength ____________________

Drug form ____________________

Usual adult dose ____________________

Amount enclosed ____________________

Prescription warning ____________________

Expiration date ____________________

Lot number ____________________

2.

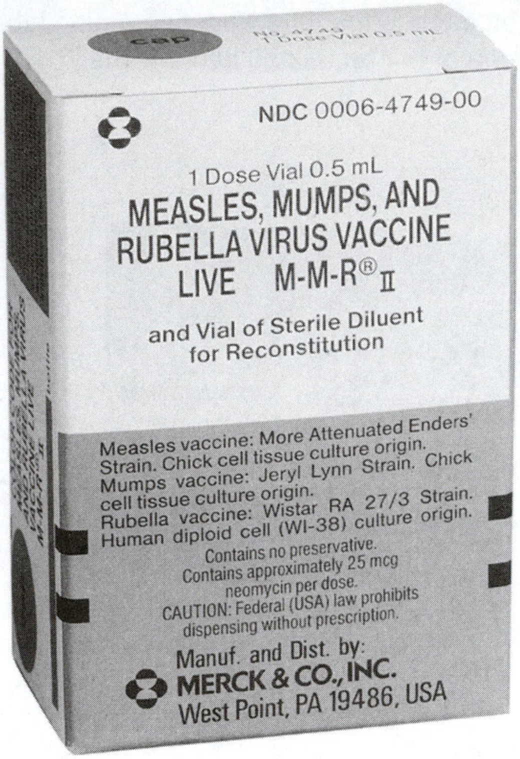

Trade name ______________________

Generic name ______________________

Manufacturer ______________________

NDC number ______________________

Dosage strength ______________________

Drug form ______________________

Usual adult dose ______________________

Amount enclosed ______________________

Prescription warning ______________________

Expiration date ______________________

Lot number ______________________

3.

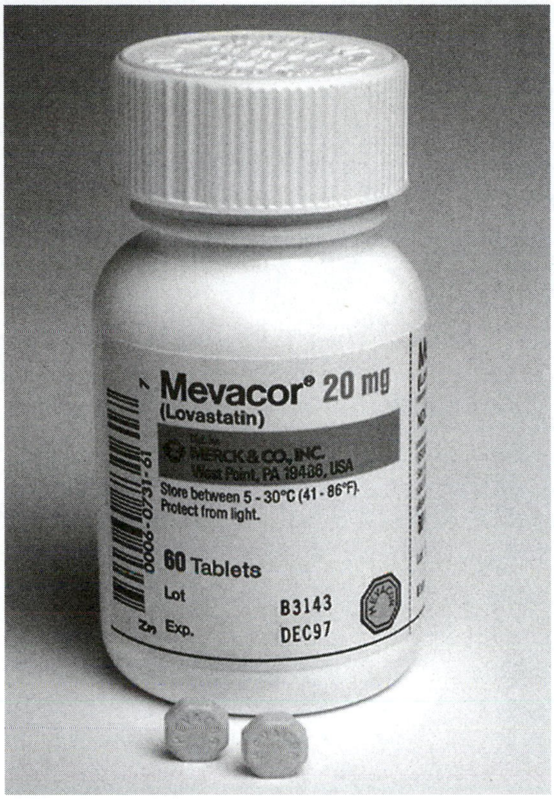

Trade name	______________
Generic name	______________
Manufacturer	______________
NDC number	______________
Dosage strength	______________
Drug form	______________
Usual adult dose	______________
Amount enclosed	______________
Prescription warning	______________
Expiration date	______________
Lot number	______________

4.

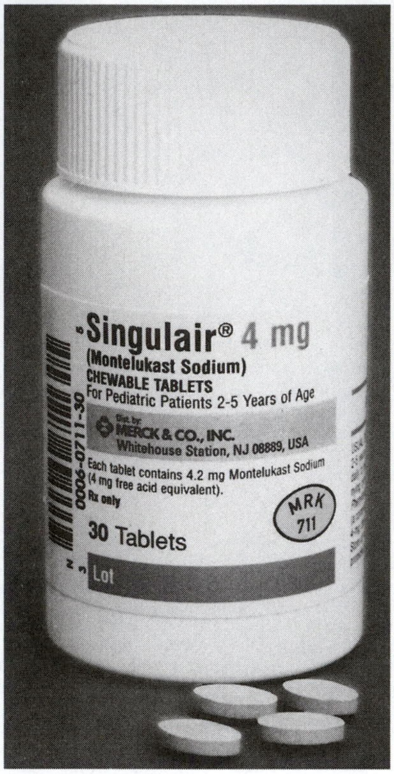

Trade name	______________
Generic name	______________
Manufacturer	______________
NDC number	______________
Dosage strength	______________
Drug form	______________
Usual adult dose	______________
Amount enclosed	______________
Prescription warning	______________
Expiration date	______________
Lot number	______________

5.

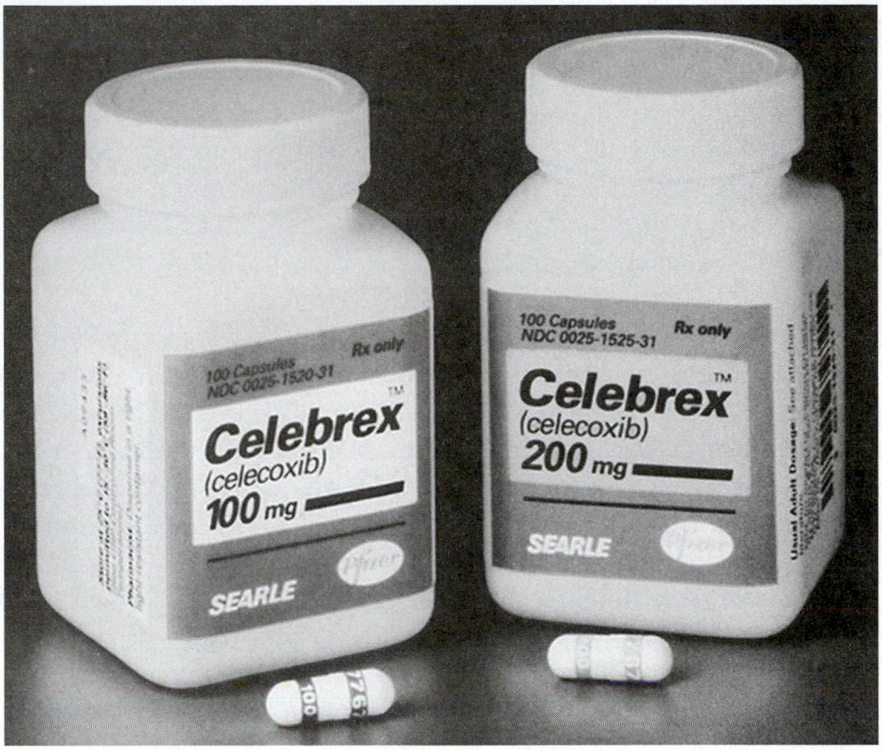

Trade name ______________________

Generic name ______________________

Manufacturer ______________________

NDC number ______________________

Dosage strength ______________________

Drug form ______________________

Usual adult dose ______________________

Amount enclosed ______________________

Prescription warning ______________________

Expiration date ______________________

Lot number ______________________

Objective

10.2 Read a medication label.

By understanding the components of a medication label, you can then read a medication label with understanding. From this label, you should be able to differentiate between the trade name and the generic name. The **trade name** is typically shown more prominently than the generic name and usually carries a ® or ™ symbol to denote a registered trademark. The **generic name** is a nonproprietary name that is used to designate a medication that is not protected by trademark.

The manufacturer's name should be apparent, as should be the NDC number. The dosage strength should be easily found and is sometimes incorporated into the trade name. Other items like the dosage strength, form, normal adult dose, and total amount enclosed should also be quite apparent. The prescription warning, which reads *CAUTION: Federal (USA) law prohibits dispensing without a prescription*, should be located on each label for prescription medications.

The **expiration date** denotes the last date in which the medication should be used. The **lot number** is an internal reference number used by the manufacturer so that medications may be traced to the day and the batch in which they were manufactured. Lot numbers are used for tracking and quality control and are vitally important should a recall occur.

SKILL SHARPENER

From the information contained on each medication label, answer the following questions.

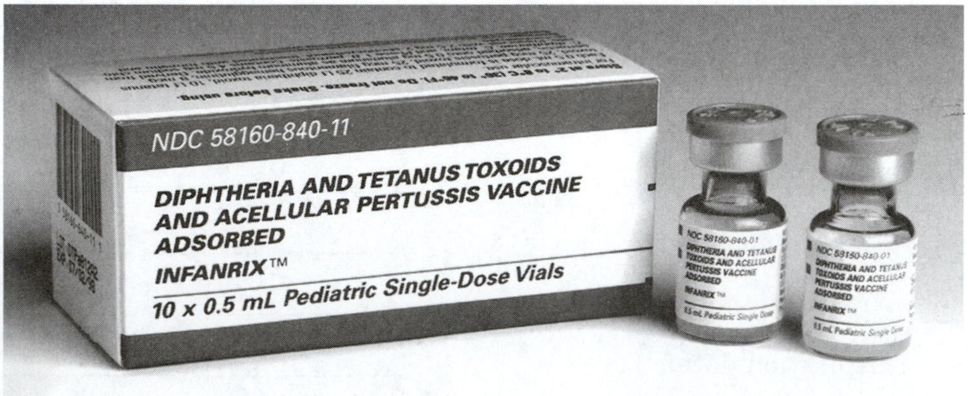

1. What is the generic name of the medication?

____

____

2. What is the trade name of the medication?

____

____

3. Are you able to see a prescription warning on this package? Why or why not?

____

____

4. What is the typical dose of this medication?

____

____

5. What is the dosage strength?

____

____

6. What is the total volume contained in this package?

____

____

7. Who is the manufacturer of this medication?

____

____

8. What is the NDC number?

____

____

9. What other components of the label should you look for?

____

____

10. What other information can you garner from reading this label?

____

____

Objective

10.3 Read a prescription.

In the same way that physicians write medication orders for patients in health care facilities, they also write prescriptions so that their patients are able to purchase medication for home use. A **prescription** is a medication order that a physician writes or telephones to the patient's local pharmacy. Like the medication label, the information must contain certain components that are common to all prescriptions (Figure 10-1). These components include:

- Physician's name, address, telephone number, and registration number
- The patient's name and address
- The date the prescription is written
- The superscription, ℞, which means take thou
- The inscription that states the name of the medication
- The subscription that gives directions for filling the prescription
- The signature, designated by the abbreviation Sig, provides directions to the patient for taking the medication

Lane Kennamer, MD
1212 Liberty Parkway • Birmingham, AL 35023
(205) 555-1438

Date ____________

Name ______________________________

Address ______________________________

℞

Generic Substitution Allowed ______________________ M.D.

Dispense As Written ______________________ M.D.

REPETATUR NR 1 2 3 p.r.n. Reg# ____________

☐ LABEL

FIGURE 10-1 Sample prescription

- Signature lines for the physician to sign indicating if a generic substitute is allowed or if the prescription must be dispensed as written
- Refill blank where the physician indicates the number of times the prescription may be refilled (by circling a number) or if no refills are allowed (designated by NR)
- A designation to the pharmacist to label the medication properly

SKILL SHARPENER

Using the prescription shown, answer the following questions.

Lane Kennamer, MD
1212 Liberty Parkway • Birmingham, AL 35023
(205) 555-1438

Date ____________

Name *Dora Reid*

Address ____________

℞ *Tussionex susp. #240 ml*
Sig 1 tsp po q 12 hr.

Generic Substitution Allowed *Lane Kennamer* M.D.

Dispense As Written ____________ M.D.

REPETATUR NR 1 (2) 3 p.r.n. Reg# ____________

☑ LABEL

1. Who is the prescribing physician?

____

____

2. What is his/her office telephone number?

____

____

3. Who is the patient?

4. What medication is prescribed?

5. What is the dosage strength of the medication?

6. How much will be dispensed?

7. Are refills prescribed?

8. Can the pharmacist offer a generic equivalent (if available)?

9. What does the symbol ℞ mean?

10. Using this mock prescription, write a concise set of instructions explaining how to take this medication, how often, and so on. Use the abbreviation list in Appendix B if necessary.

Objective

10.4 Read a syringe.

Syringes are used to administer precise amounts of medication, either through injections into the skin or muscle or through infusions into an intravenous line. Marked with a series of graduations to indicate volume, syringes come in a variety of sizes, but are read in the same manner. The syringe should be read at the edge of the plunger nearest the needle. This point indicates the remaining volume of solution in the syringe.

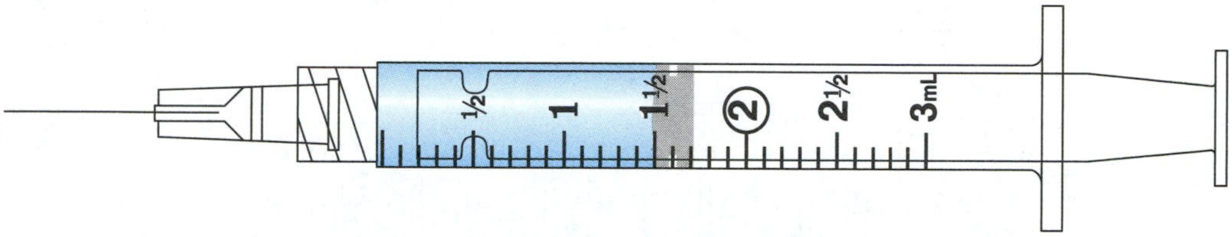

In this example, there is 1 1/2 mL remaining in the syringe. Assuming the syringe started with 3 mL, 1 1/2 mL has been administered.

SKILL SHARPENER

Determine the amount of solution remaining in each of the following syringes.

1. ______________________________

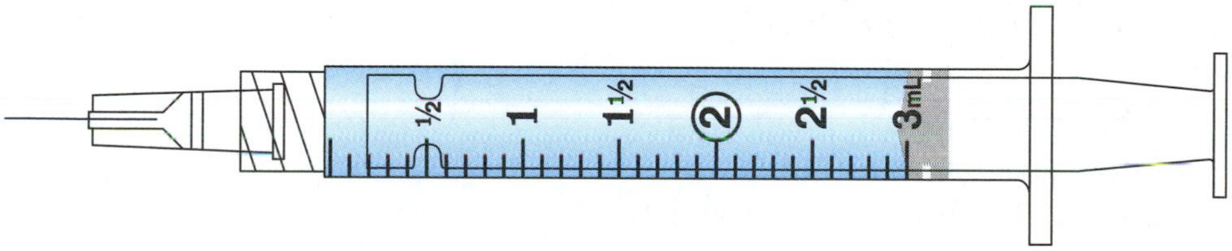

2. ______________________________

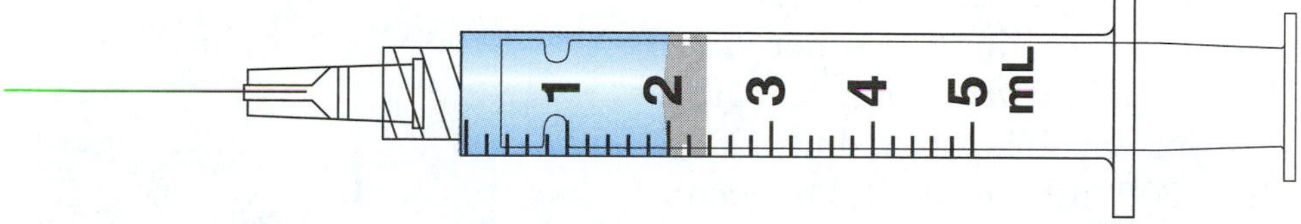

3. ______________________________

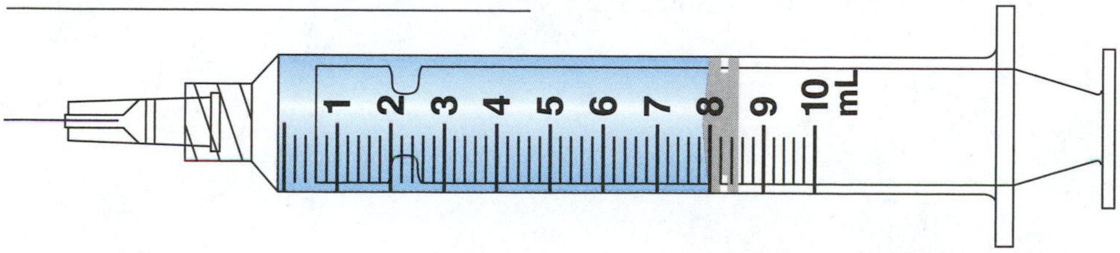

4. ______________________________

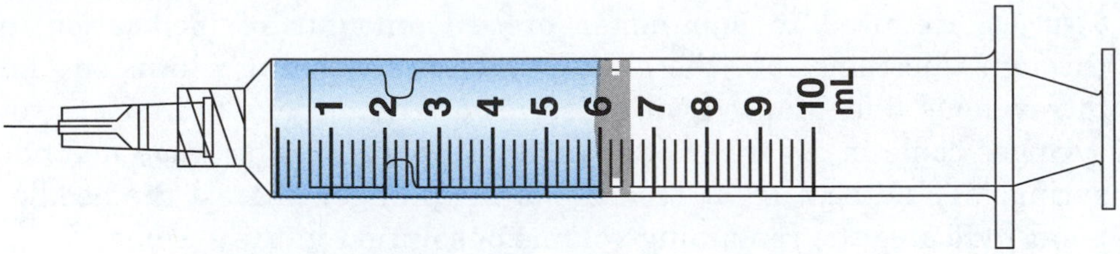

5. ______________________________

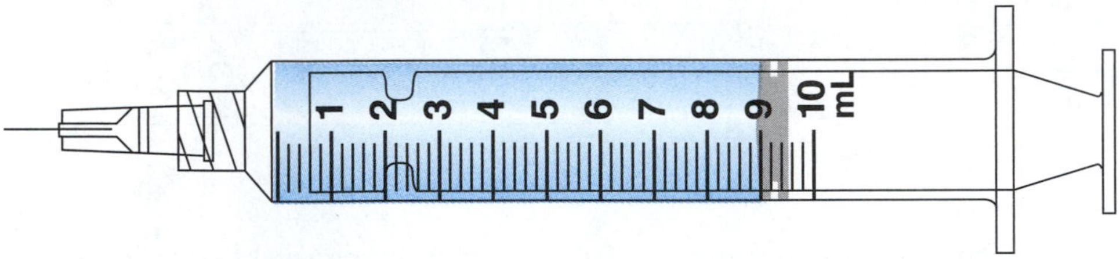

Objective

10.5 Determine the amount of fluid remaining in an intravenous bag.

Intravenous fluids come in both glass bottles and plastic bags. To measure the amount of fluid infused, note the level of the fluid. The marking that is even with the top of the fluid solution will tell you the amount of fluid remaining. To determine how much fluid has been infused, subtract the fluid remaining from the capacity of the bag.

IV bags are commonly supplied as 250 mL, 500 mL, or 1,000 mL. Smaller bags of 100 mL are available to mix certain medications. Check the capacity of the IV bag by noting the capacity displayed on the bag.

The bag illustrated here is a 1,000 mL bag. Also, note that the current level is at 2, indicating that 200 mL of fluid has been infused and 800 mL remains.

1,000 mL − 200 mL = 800 mL

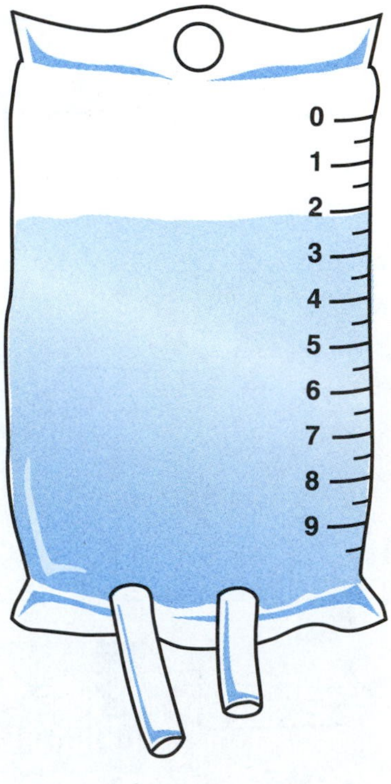

SKILL SHARPENER

Indicate both the volume remaining and the amount infused in each of the following examples.

1. Volume remaining: ______________

Amount infused: ______________

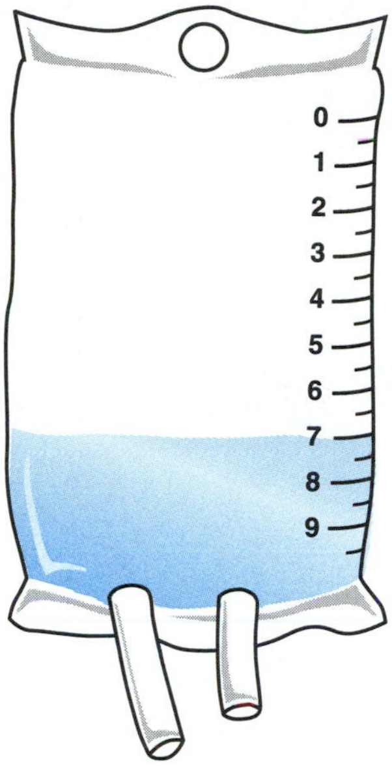

2. Volume remaining: ______________

Amount infused: ______________

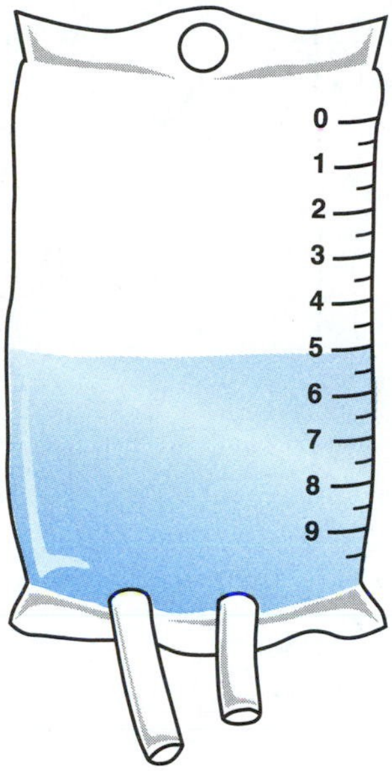

3. Volume remaining: ______________

Amount infused: ______________

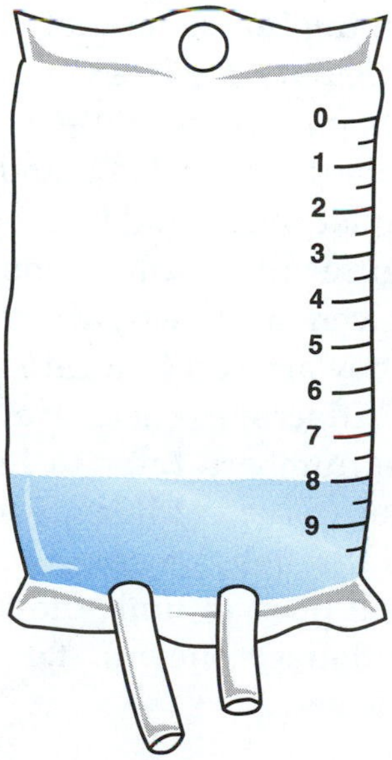

4. Volume remaining: ______________

Amount infused: ______________

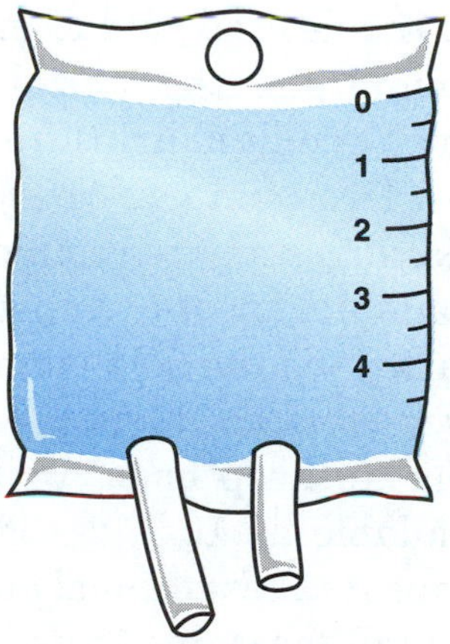

5. Volume remaining: ____________

Amount infused: ____________

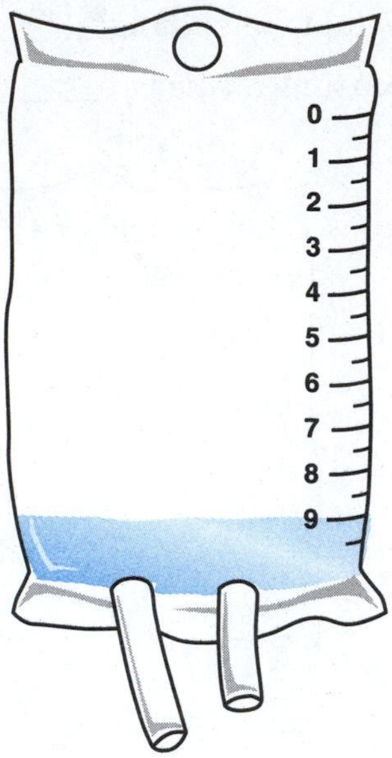

Objective

10.6 Calculate intravenous drip rates.

The rate of intravenous fluid infusions is controlled by either gravity-fed hand controls or electronic pumps. Electronic pumps require only that you set the desired rate of infusion. When controlling infusions that are not on a pump, a mathematical formula is used to calculate **drip rates**, or the rate in which the fluid drips from the IV bag into the intravenous line.

Two common types of drip sets exist. Sometimes called standard sets, **macrodrip** sets are commonly used for fluid replacement and to keep a route available for intravenous medications (Figure 10-2). Intravenous lines, started for the sole purpose of assuring intravenous access, are sometimes referred to as **TKO lines** or **KVO lines** because they are run at a rate sufficient only "to keep open" or to "keep vein open." Macrodrip sets are typically available as 10-, 12-, or 15-drop sets. These numbers refer to how many drops it takes to equal one mL of fluid. In other words, a 15-drop set delivers one mL for every 15 drops of fluid that drips through the set.

A **microdrip** set is utilized when there is a need to limit the volume of fluid infused (Figure 10-3). Microdrip sets deliver one mL for every 60 (smaller) drops of fluid that drips through the set.

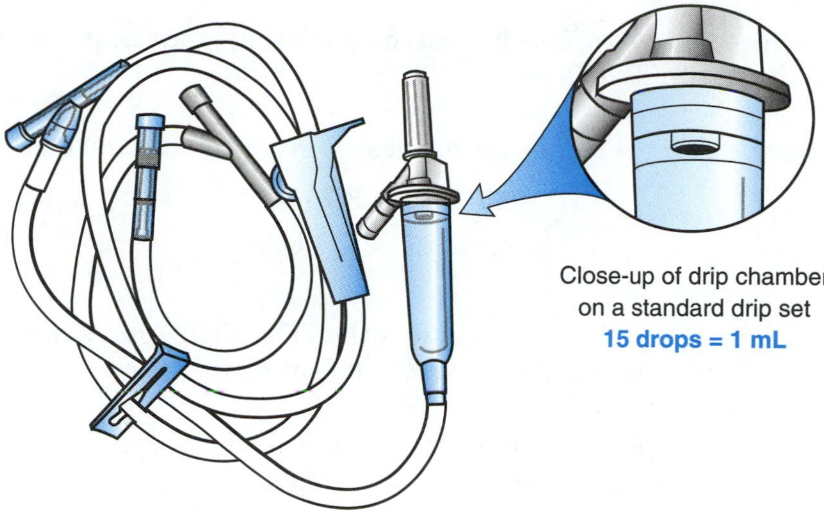

FIGURE 10-2 A macrodrip set is sometimes referred to as a standard set.

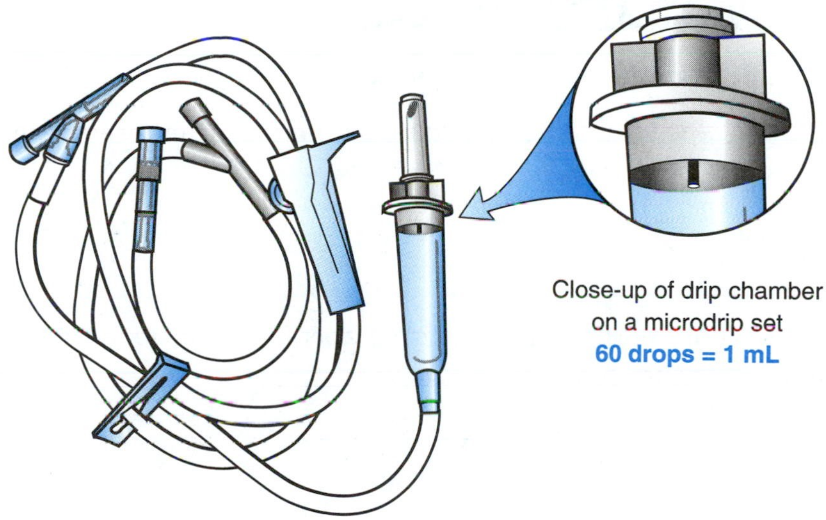

FIGURE 10-3 A microdrip set is sometimes referred to as a minidrip set.

The following formula is used to determine how to adjust the drip set to administer the desired amount of fluid over the prescribed time.

amount to be infused × drip set ÷ time of infusion (in minutes) = number of drops per minute to be infused

Example

You are asked to infuse 250 mL over 3 hours. Your hospital uses a 15-drop-per-mL drip set.

amount × drip set ÷ time (in minutes) = drops per minute to be infused

$$250 \times 15 = 3{,}750$$

$$3{,}750 \div 180 = 20.8\overline{33}$$

Therefore, you will need to adjust the IV to drip approximately once every three seconds to deliver 250 mL in three hours.

When a constant infusion of medication is given over time, **piggyback** infusions may be used. A piggyback is a secondary infusion that is attached to an already existing (primary) IV line. The primary line is turned off and the piggybacked line delivers the necessary infusion of medication.

SKILL SHARPENER

Figure the drip rate for the following scenarios.

1. You are asked to administer 1,000 mL of normal saline over 24 hours using a 15-drop-per-mL set.

   ____

2. You need to adjust the flow rate of an existing IV line to administer 200 mL over 1 1/2 hours. A 10-drop set is used.

   ____

3. You need to administer 350 mL of lactated ringers over 180 minutes using a 12-drop set.

   ____

4. Figure how to administer 500 mL of normal saline over 2 hours using a 15-drop set.

   ____

5. Using a 15-drop set, administer 100 mL of saline over 30 minutes.

   ____

Objective

10.7 Determine the concentration of solutions.

A *solution* is a liquid that has another substance, such as medication or minerals, dissolved in it. The substance that is dissolved in the liquid is called the *solute*. The liquid is called the *solvent*.

The **concentration of a solution** refers to the amount of the solute that has been dissolved in a specific amount of liquid. Concentrations are frequently noted by the use of percentages.

Example

If 2 parts of a mineral are placed in 100 parts of liquid, the concentration of the solution is 2:100. This could also be noted as 2/100, 0.02, or 2%.

SKILL SHARPENER

Indicate the ratio of solute to solvent in the following, first by using a ratio (x:100) and then by converting to a percentage (x%).

1. 4 parts of drug in 100 parts of liquid ________ :100 ________ %
2. 12.5 parts of a mineral in 100 parts of liquid ________ :100 ________ %
3. 50 parts of glucose in 100 parts water ________ :100 ________ %
4. 10 parts of glucose in 100 parts water ________ :100 ________ %
5. 9 parts of sodium chloride in 100 parts water ________ :100 ________ %

PERCENT STRENGTH

Percent strength refers to the percentage of solvent in a given solute. For instance, if the medication order is for 10 mL of a 25% solution, first realize that the 25% refers to 25 parts of 100, noted as 25:100. Since you must give 10 mL of the solution, use proportions to figure how much of the drug or mineral would be mixed with the fluid to yield the desired solution.

The problem: You are asked to administer 10 mL of a 25% solution.

Set up as:

$$25 : 100 :: x : 10$$

(25 : 100 — Refers to 25% solution; x — Grams of drug; 10 — 10 mL ordered)

Multiply the means. $25 : 100 :: x : 10$

$$100 \times x = 100x$$

Multiply the extremes. $25 : 100 :: x : 10$

$$25 \times 10 = 250$$

Set up as:

$$100x = 250$$

To solve for x, divide 100 into both sides.

$$100x \div 100 = 1x \text{ or } x$$

$$250 \div 100 = 2.5$$

Solution: $x = 2.5$

Therefore, mix 2.5 grams of drug in 10 mL to yield a 25% solution.

SKILL SHARPENER

How much of the solvent (drug or mineral) must be given to attain the following solutions? Figure using proportions and show your work.

1. 10 mL of a 6% solution ______________________

2. 75 mL of a 9% solution ______________________

3. 15 mL of a 35% solution ______________________

4. 150 mL of a 10% solution ______________________

5. 120 mL of a 0.9% solution. ______________________

Objective

10.8 Calculate medication dosages using proportions.

Every day, health care professionals calculate medication dosages in an effort to administer the correct amount of medication for the best therapeutic effect. Though there are a number of ways that medication doses are figured, proportions will be used here. By using critical thinking skills, proportions will help you to solve a vast number of problems.

The problem:

You are asked to administer 40 mg of furosemide.
It is packaged 10 mg/mL in an 8 mL ampule.

Set up as:

40 mg : x mL : : 10 mg : 1 mL

Multiply the means. 40 : x : : 10 : 1

$x \times 10 = 10x$

Multiply the extremes. 40 : x : : 10 : 1

$40 \times 1 = 40$

Set up as:

$10x = 40$

To solve for x, divide both sides by 10.

$10x \div 10 = 1x$ or x

$40 \div 10 = 4$

Solution: $x = 4$ mL

Therefore, administer 4 mL to deliver 40 mg of furosemide.

SKILL SHARPENER

In each of the following problems, use proportions to determine the volume of medication to be given.

1. You are asked to administer 60 mg of furosemide. It is packaged 10 mg/mL in an 8 mL ampule. How many mL do you administer?

   ____

2. Administer 0.65 mg of dexamethasone elixir. It is packaged 0.5 mg/mL. How many mL do you administer?

   ____

3. Lidocaine is available in an ampule with 100 mg in 5 mL of solution. How many mL do you give to administer 65 mg?

   ____

4. Lorazepam is supplied 2 mg/mL in a 1 mL vial. You need to administer 3 mg slow IV. How many mL do you give?

   ____

5. Lovastatin is supplied in 20 mg tablets. You are asked to administer 60 mg. How many tablets do you give?

   ____

6. Lovenox is packaged 120 mg/0.8 mL. How many mL do you give to administer 40 mg?

   ____

7. Compazine is supplied 10 mg in a 2 mL vial. How many mL do you give to administer 2.5 mg?

   ____

8. Tenormin is supplied 5 mg in 10 mL ampules. How may mL do you give to administer 5 mg?

____

9. You are called upon to administer 8 units Pitocin. It is supplied in a 1 mL ampule that contains 10 units. How many mL do you administer?

____

10. You need to administer 1 mg of epinephrine. It is packaged 10 mg/10 mL. How many mL do you administer?

____

Objective

10.9 Convert medication dosages for home use.

Patients sometimes have to take medications at home. Health care professionals may be called upon to instruct patients how to convert measurements from the metric or apothecary system to the household system. For instance, a patient may be asked to take 5 mL of a cough elixir. As a health care professional, you should be able to instruct him or her to take 1 teaspoon (tsp) as an approximate equivalent.

The ability to assist patients in this way depends on:

- knowing metric/apothecary/household equivalents.
- being able to use proportions to make conversions as necessary.
- knowing the necessary terminology and abbreviations.

A listing of common abbreviations is included in Appendix B and equivalencies are noted in Appendix C.

SKILL SHARPENER

Using the household system of measurement, clearly write how much and how often the patient should take the medicine. Use Appendix B and Appendix C if necessary.

1. The prescription calls for the patient to take 15 mL of a cough syrup PO b.i.d.

2. The order calls for 1 fldr of an elixir PO q.i.d.

3. Instruct the patient to take 25 mg PO q 4 hours prn nausea. The medicine is supplied in 25 mg tablets.

4. The patient should take 240 mg PO qd until gone. The prescription says to dispense #14, 120 mg capsules.

5. Take 1/150 gr SL prn chest pain. This medication comes packaged in 0.4 mg tablets.

6. The doctor wants the patient to take gr ss PO t.i.d. The tablets are 10 mg.

7. The doctor orders 0.5 g to take PO b.i.d. The capsules come in 250 mg strength.

____

____

____

8. The patient must drink a substance before a test the following day. The patient should take 240 mL PO HS, then should be NPO until after the test.

____

____

____

9. The patient should take 1 oz of medication PO pc.

____

____

____

10. Direct the patient to take 2 dr PO q.o.d.

____

____

____

CONCLUSION

Medication administration is an important responsibility that should not be taken lightly. Health care professionals must assure that patients receive the intended dose of the correct medicine by carefully interpreting orders, accurately calculating dosages, and unfalteringly administering the intended medication.

Attention to detail is imperative. Erroneously moving the decimal one place in either direction could result in administering one tenth or ten times the desired dose of a drug. Though calculating medication dosages may be a routine part of a typical day, the health care professional must remain alert and diligent to ensure accuracy.

REVIEW AND REFLECT

1. Why is it important to carefully control the flow of intravenous fluids?

2. Why is it important to be able to instruct patients how to take medications using household measurements?

3. Describe the importance of precision in reading prescriptions.

4. Why is important to know how to determine the concentration of solutions?

5. Why do you think that medication labels and prescriptions have standardized components?

CHAPTER 11

Weights and Measures

LEARNING OBJECTIVES

After completing this chapter, the reader will be able to:

- **11.1** Read scales.
- **11.2** Convert between English and metric weight measurements.
- **11.3** Read an English (household) ruler.
- **11.4** Read a metric ruler.
- **11.5** Convert between English and metric length measurements.
- **11.6** Read a thermometer.
- **11.7** Convert between Fahrenheit and Celsius.
- **11.8** Determine body surface area.

MATH IN THE REAL WORLD

"Since some medications are dosed based upon weight, we have to estimate the patient's weight...[we] sometimes use measurements as simple as how many inches of nitroglycerine paste the patient uses."

Roger G. Wootten, AAS, EMT-Paramedic

KEY TERMS

- body surface area (BSA)
- Celsius
- Fahrenheit
- nomogram

SELF-ASSESSMENT **PRETEST**

Read the following scales.

1. ______________________________

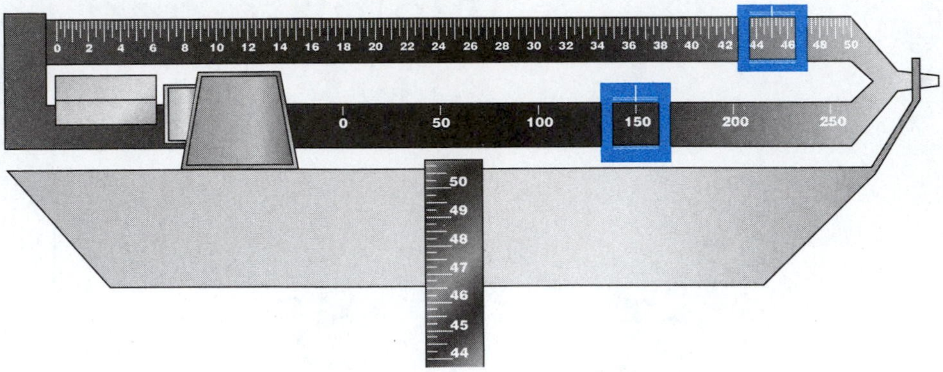

2. ______________________________

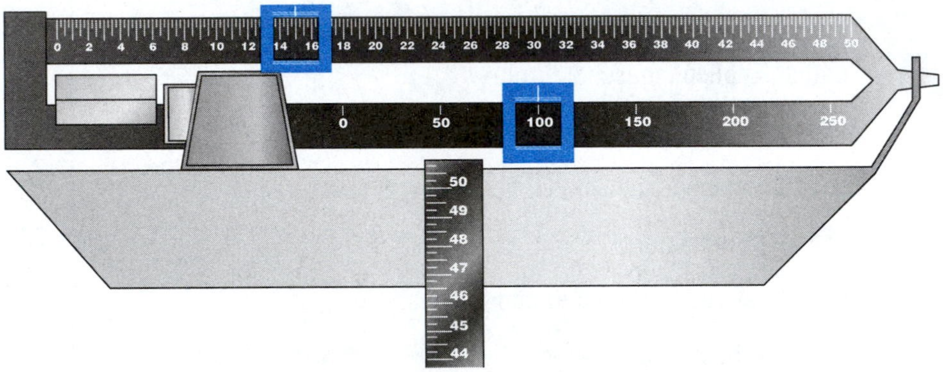

3. ______________________________

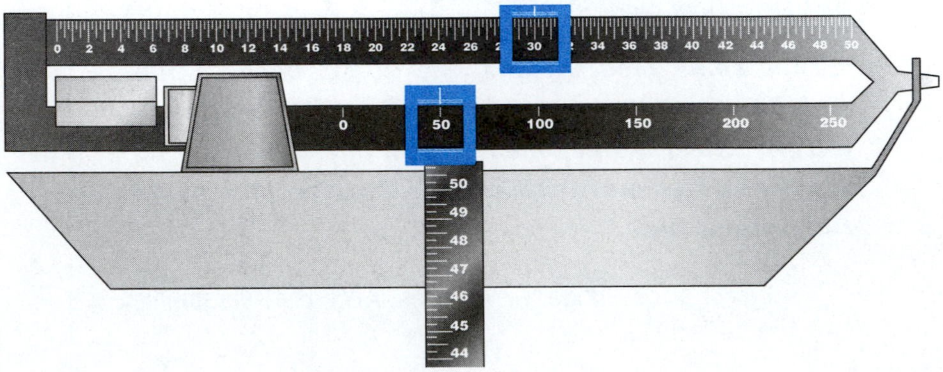

4. ______________________

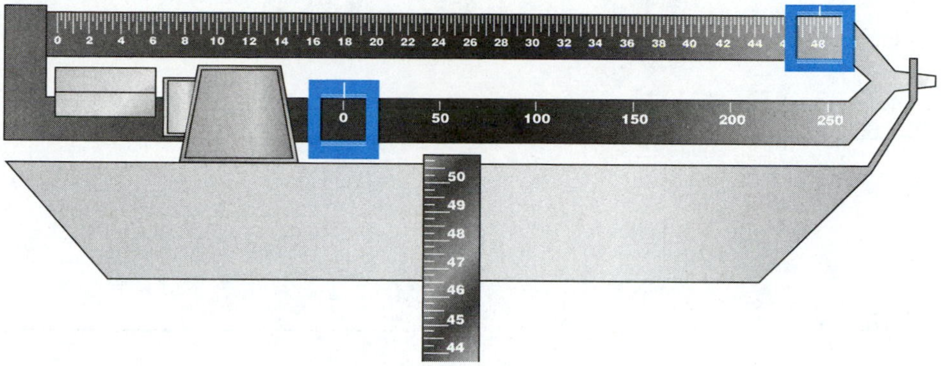

5. ______________________

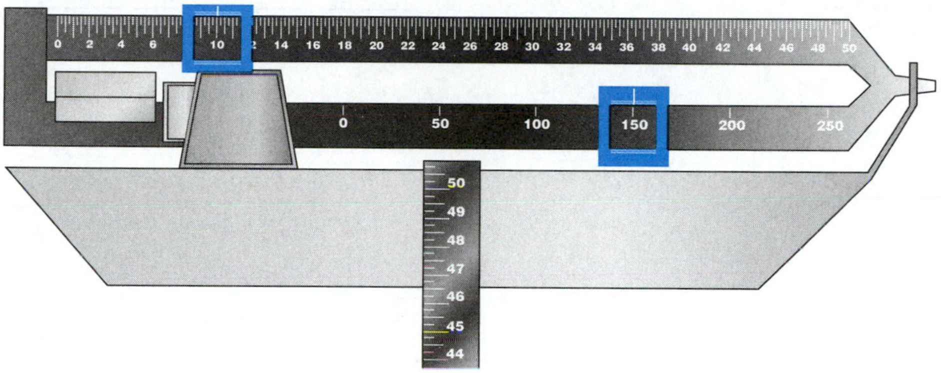

Convert the following weights to kilograms.

6. 150 lb ______________________

7. 222 lb ______________________

8. 25 lb ______________________

9. 39 lb ______________________

10. 165 lb ______________________

11. 155 lb ______________________

12. 249 lb ______________________

13. 12 lb ______________________

14. 2 lb ______________________

15. 6 lb ______________________

Convert kilograms to pounds.

16. 68 kg ______________________

17. 9 kg ______________________

18. 324 kg ____________________

19. 75 kg ____________________

20. 91 kg ____________________

21. 100 kg ____________________

22. 12 kg ____________________

23. 29 kg ____________________

24. 66 kg ____________________

25. 128 kg ____________________

212

Record the lengths indicated on the following rulers.

26. ______________________

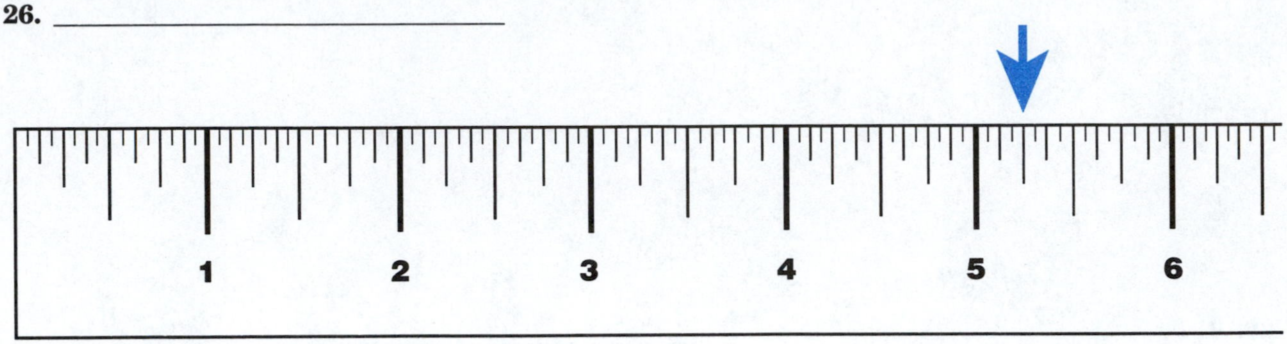

27. ______________________

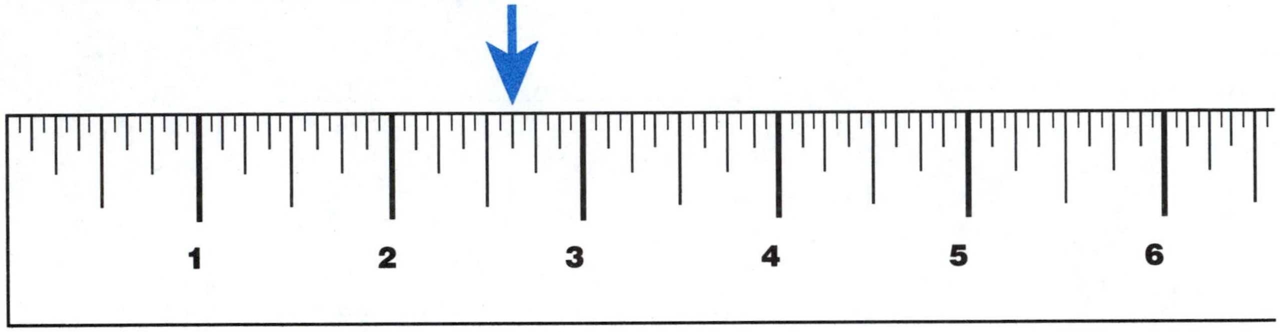

28. ______________________

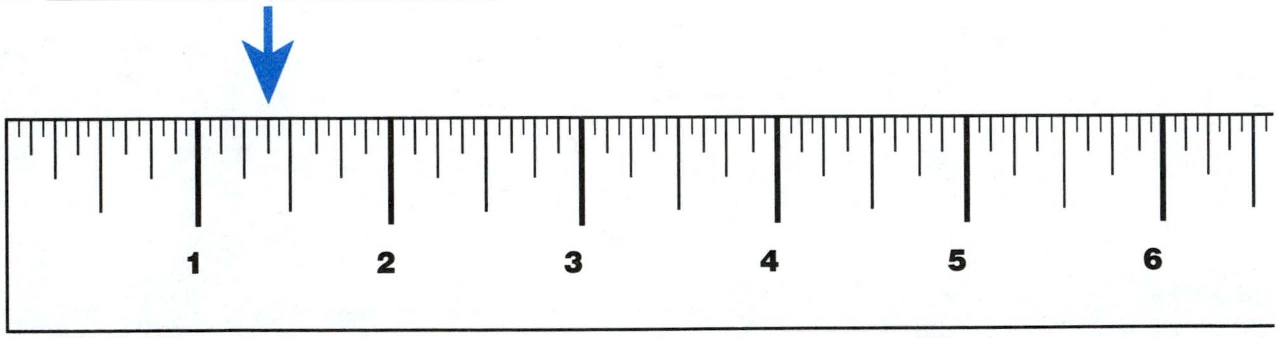

29. ______________________

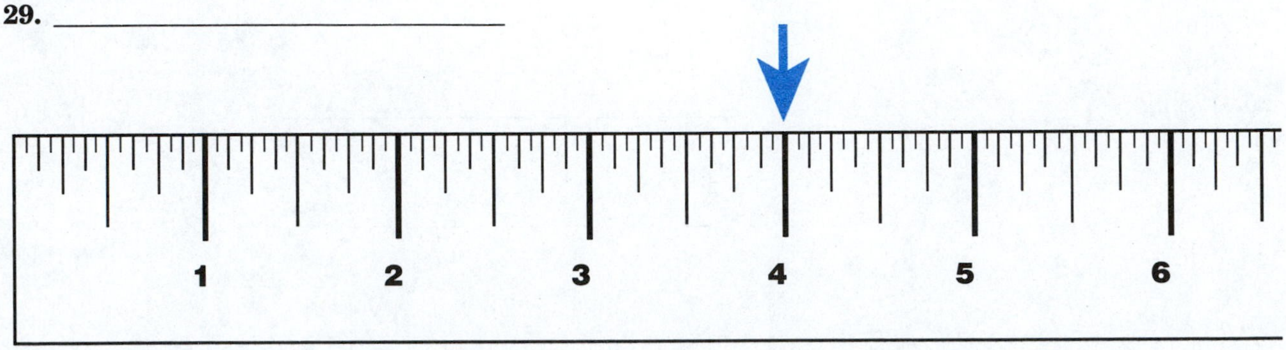

30. ______________________________

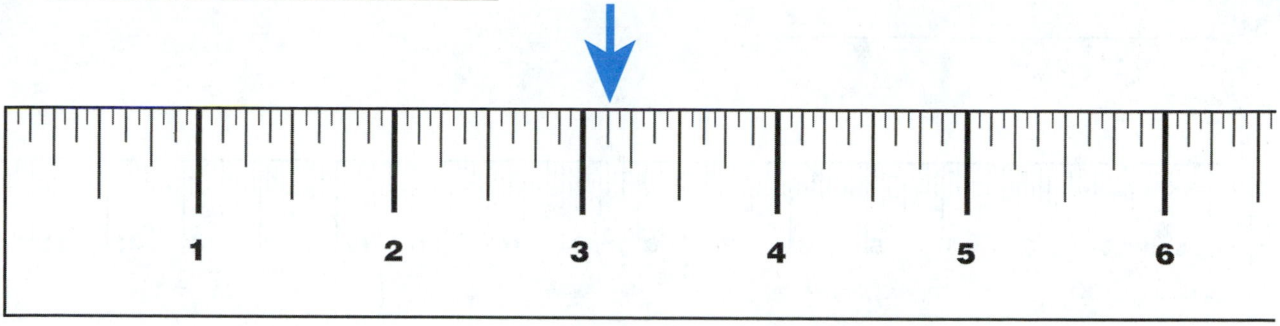
1
2
3
4
5
6

31. ______________________________

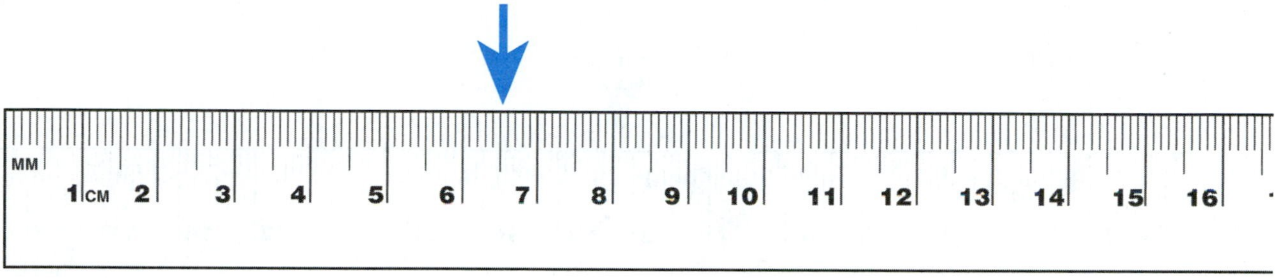
MM
1 CM
2
3
4
5
6
7
8
9
10
11
12
13
14
15
16

32. ______________________________

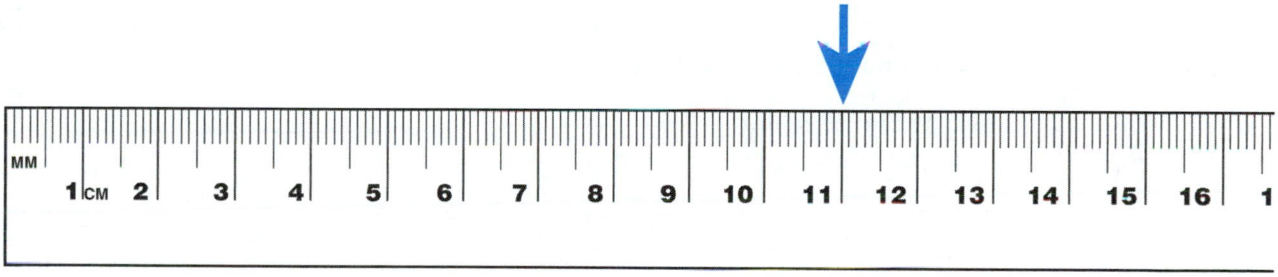
MM
1 CM
2
3
4
5
6
7
8
9
10
11
12
13
14
15
16
1

33. ______________________________

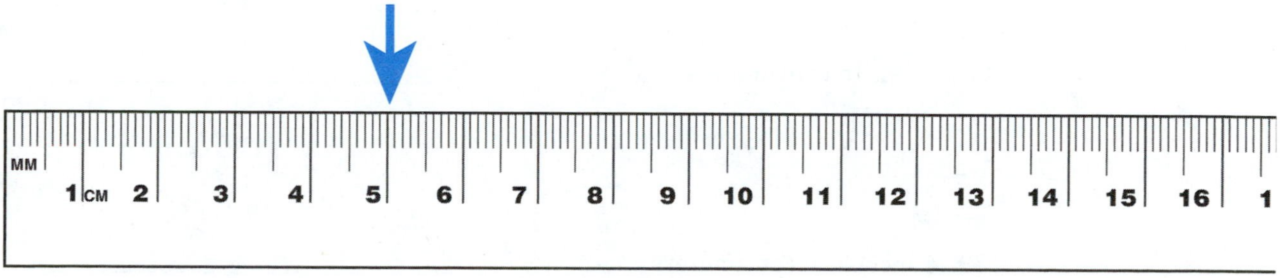
MM
1 CM
2
3
4
5
6
7
8
9
10
11
12
13
14
15
16
1

34. ______________________________

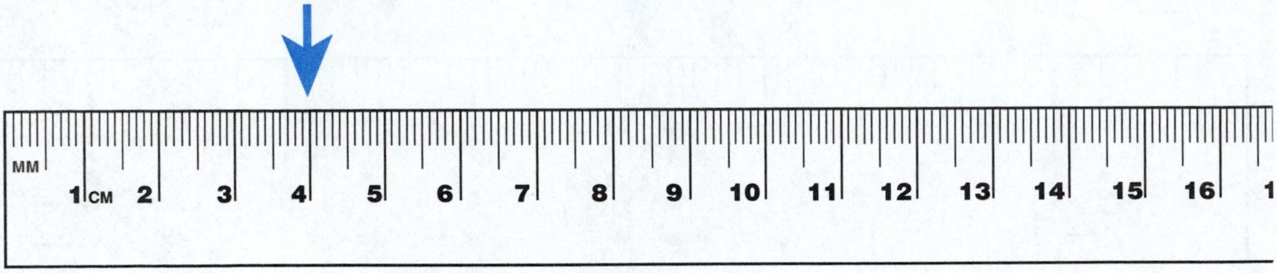

35. ______________________________

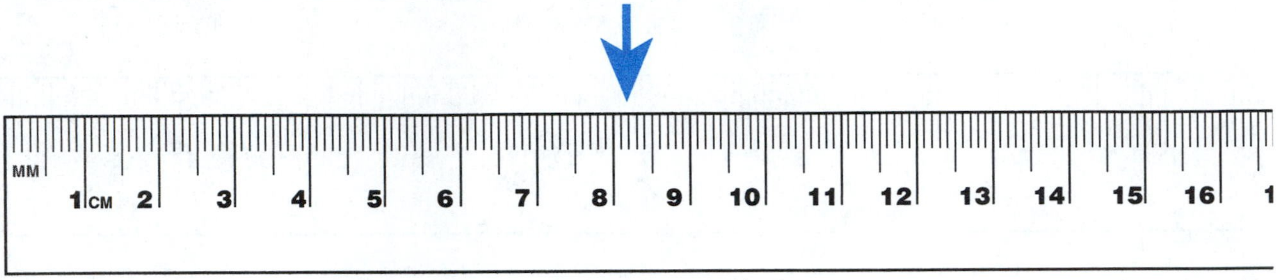

Convert the following English length measurements to metric length measurements as directed.

36. 17 feet to meters ______________________________

37. 9 yards to meters ______________________________

38. 6 feet to centimeters ______________________________

39. 4 inches to centimeters ______________________________

40. 2 1/2 inches to millimeters ______________________

41. 76 inches to centimeters ______________________

42. 8 feet to centimeters ______________________

43. 14.5 feet to centimeters ______________________

44. 12.5 feet to meters ______________________

45. 99 feet to meters ______________________

Convert metric length measurements to English length measurements.

46. 3 meters to feet ______________________

47. 12 meters to feet ______________________

48. 33 meters to feet ______________________

49. 45 cm to inches ______________________

50. 575 mm to inches ______________________

51. 9,080 mm to inches ______________________

52. 55 mm to inches ______________________

53. 655 meters to yards ______________________

54. 8,500 cm to feet ______________________

55. 1,275 mm to inches ______________________

Read the temperatures on the following thermometers.

56. ______________________

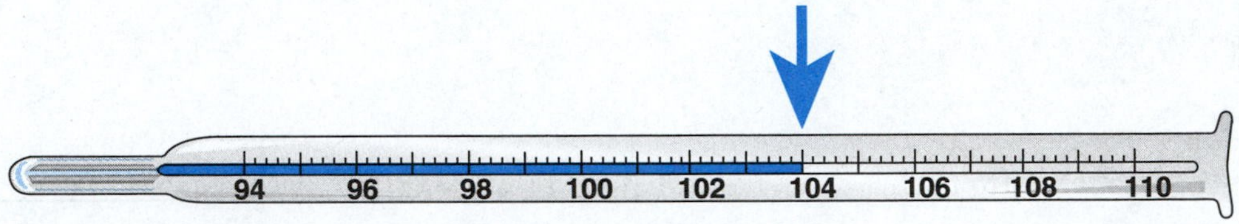

57. ______________________________

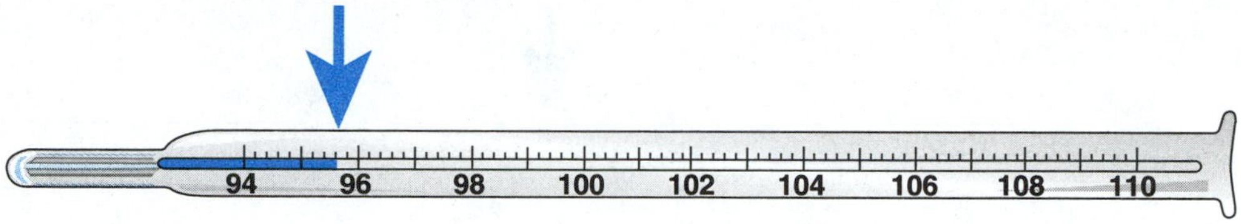

58. ______________________________

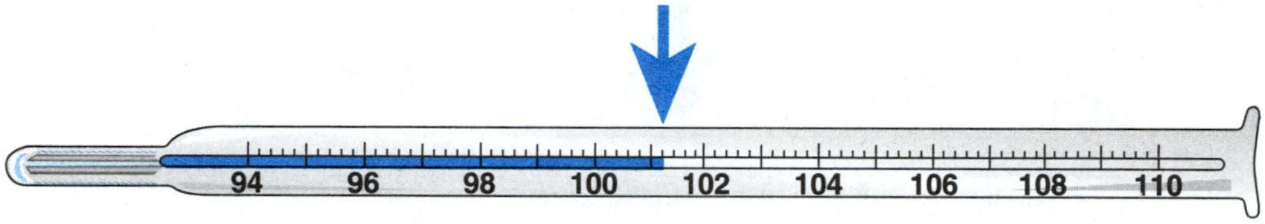

59. ______________________________

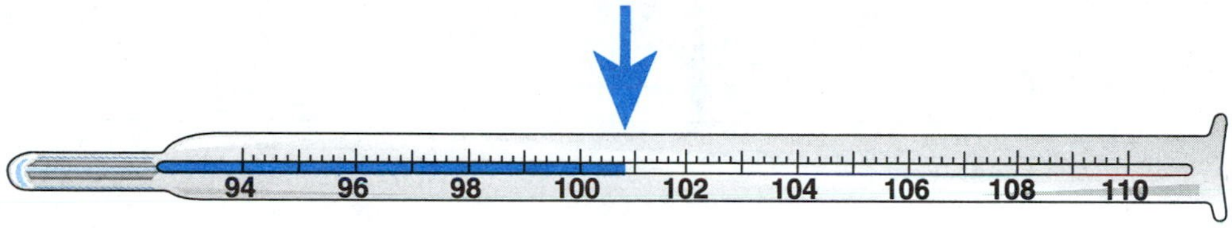

60. ______________________________

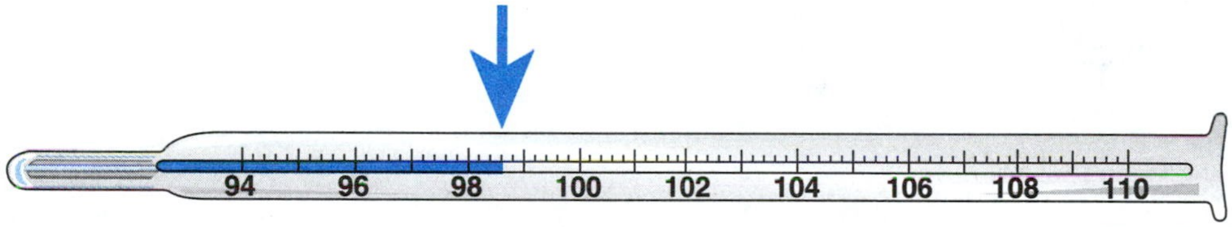

61. ______________________________

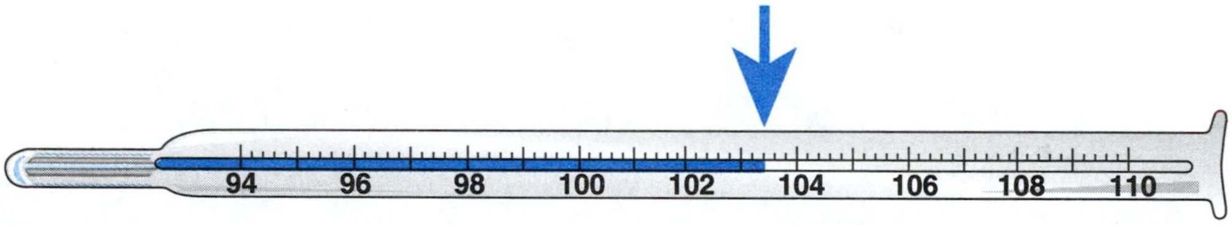

62. ______________________________

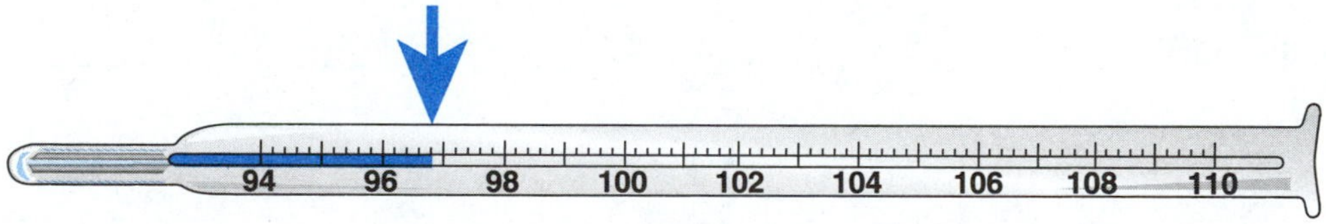

63. ______________________

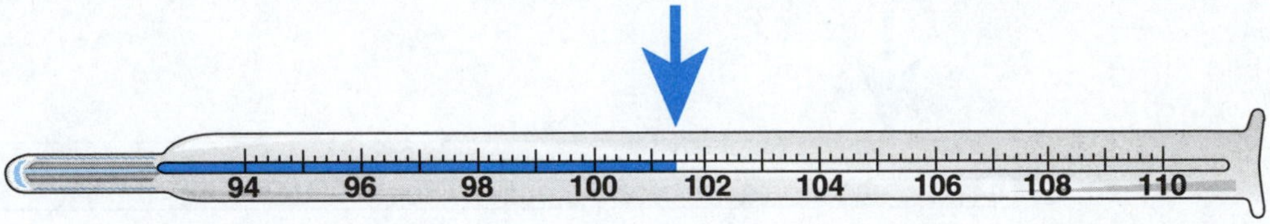

64. ______________________

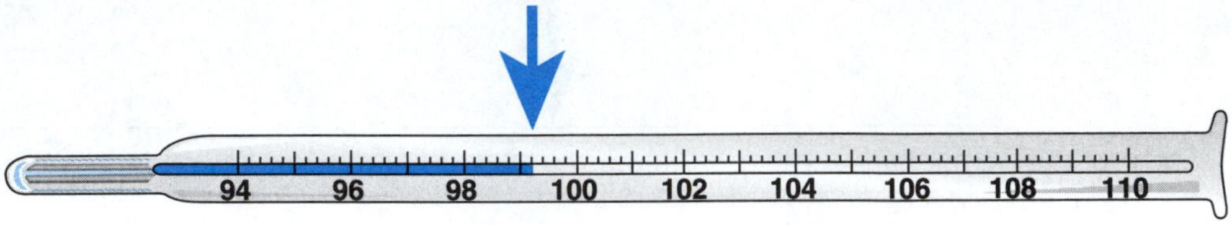

65. ______________________

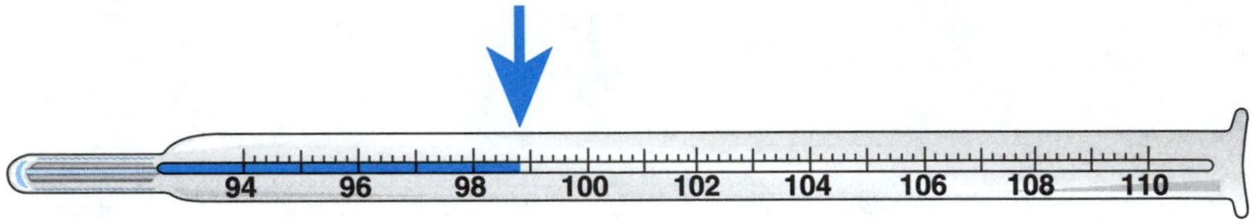

Convert the following temperatures from Fahrenheit to Celsius.

66. 98.6°F ______________________

67. 78°F ______________________

68. 102°F ______________________

69. 55°F ______________________

70. 1,250°F ______________________

71. 212°F ______________________

72. 325°F ______________________

73. 450°F ______________________

74. 900°F ______________________

75. 1°F ______________________

Convert the following temperatures from Celsius to Fahrenheit.

76. 12°C ______________________

77. 34°C ______________________

78. 55°C ______________________

79. 22°C ______________________

80. 118°C ______________________

81. 123°C ______________________

82. 234°C ______________________

83. 90°C ______________________

84. 23°C ______________________

85. 132°C ______________________

Determine the estimated body surface area (BSA) for the following patients.

86. 35-lb child of normal height for her weight

____

87. 7-lb infant of normal height for his weight

____

88. 60-lb child of normal height for her weight

____

89. 71-inch patient who weighs 80 kg

____

90. 50-cm patient who weighs 5 kg

____

INTRODUCTION

Health care professionals may need to convert English and metric measures. This includes converting from yards, feet, and inches to meters, centimeters, and millimeters and from Fahrenheit to Celsius and Celsius to Fahrenheit. This chapter will introduce the concepts necessary to perform these operations.

Objective

11.1 Read scales.

Since some medication dosages are determined based on weight, it is important for health care professionals to accurately read scales and record weights. Read the scale as explained in Figure 11-1.

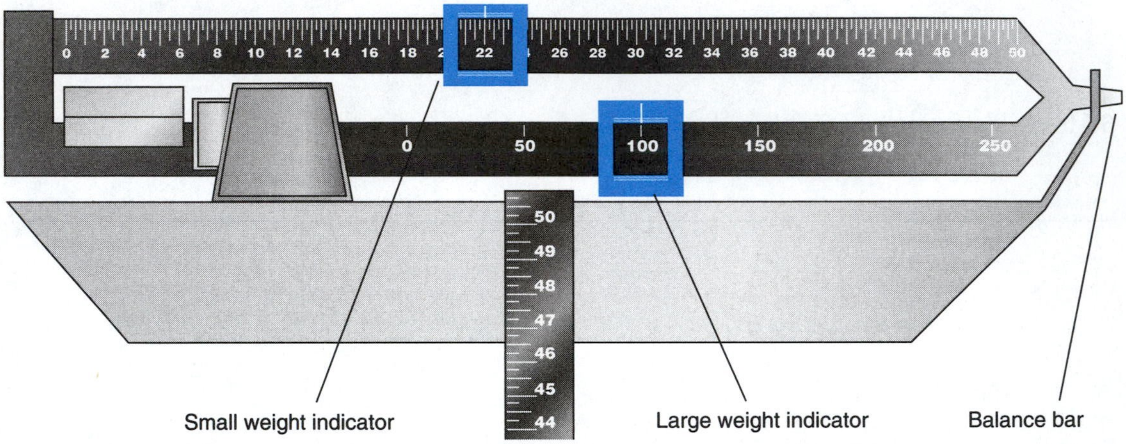

FIGURE 11-1 The weight shown on the upper and lower bars are added for the total weight.

SKILL SHARPENER

Read the following scales.

1. ______________________________

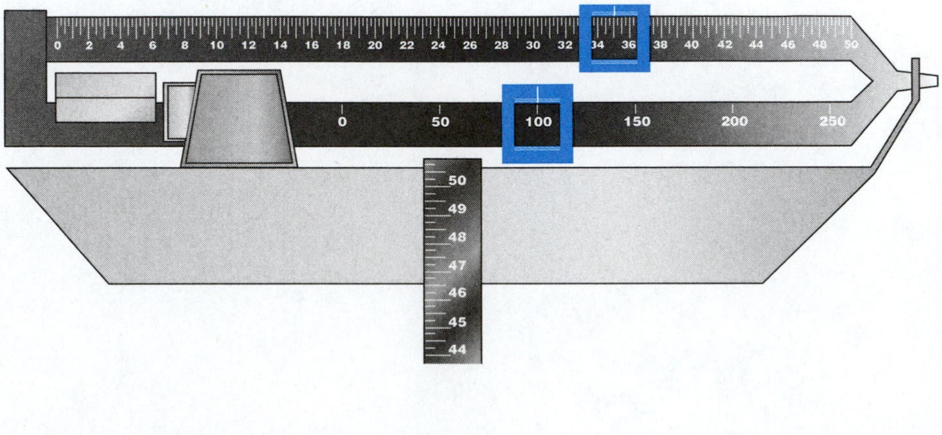

2. ______________________________

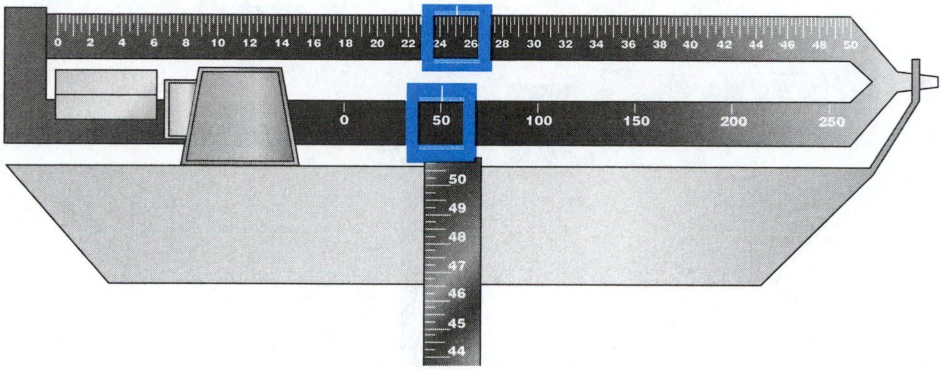
0 2 4 6 8 10 12 14 16 18 20 22 24 26 28 30 32 34 36 38 40 42 44 46 48 50
0 50 100 150 200 250
50 49 48 47 46 45 44

3. ______________________________

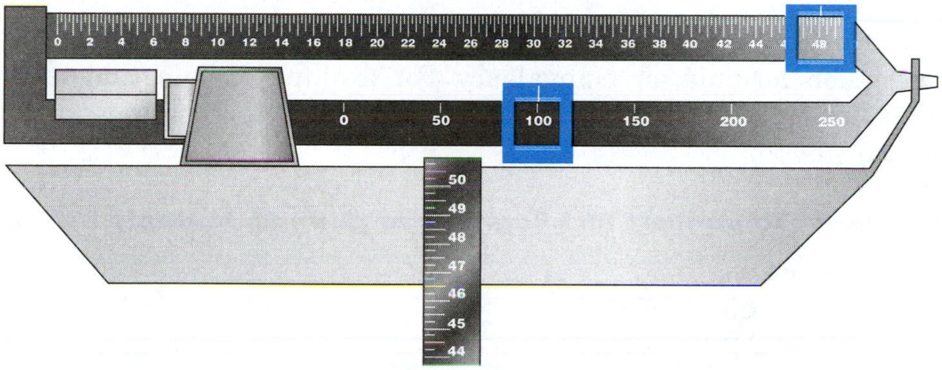
0 2 4 6 8 10 12 14 16 18 20 22 24 26 28 30 32 34 36 38 40 42 44 48
0 50 100 150 200 250
50 49 48 47 46 45 44

4. ______________________________

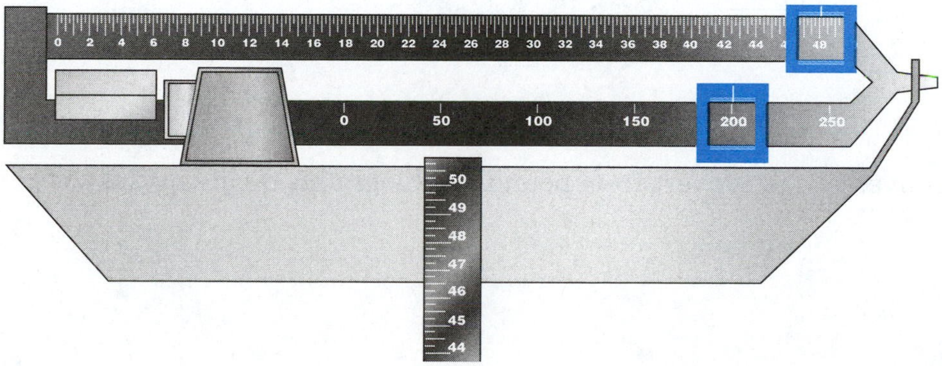
0 2 4 6 8 10 12 14 16 18 20 22 24 26 28 30 32 34 36 38 40 42 44 48
0 50 100 150 200 250
50 49 48 47 46 45 44

5. ________________________

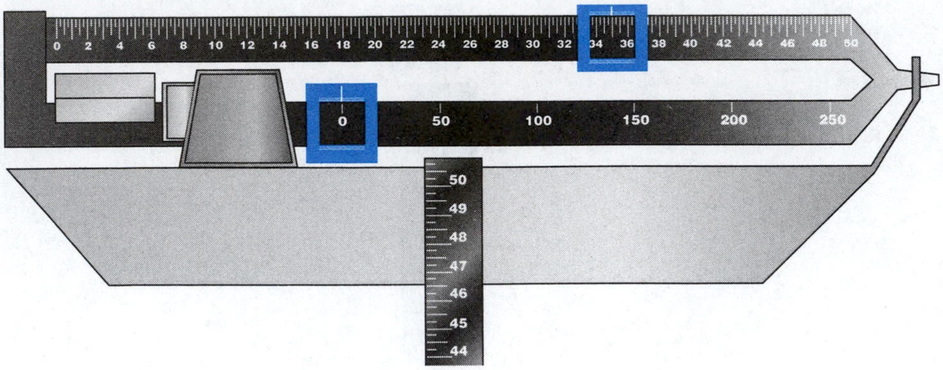

Objective

11.2 Convert between English and metric weight measurements.

To convert from English to metric weight measurements you must know the conversion formula, or equivalency. For example, 1 kilogram is roughly equivalent to 2.2 pounds. When converting from kilograms to pounds, multiply by 2.2.

Example: To convert 65 kilograms to pounds, multiply by 2.2.

Set up as:

$$\begin{array}{r} 65 \\ \underline{\times\ 2.2} \end{array}$$

Multiply.

$$\begin{array}{r} 65 \\ \underline{\times\ 2.2} \\ 130 \\ \underline{130} \\ 143.0 \end{array}$$

Solution: 65 kg = 143 lb

Conversely, to convert from pounds to kilograms, divide by 2.2.

Example: To convert 165 pounds to kilograms, divide by 2.2.

Set up as:

$$2.2\overline{)165}$$

Move decimals to right.

$$2.2\overline{)165.0}$$

Divide.

```
      75.
22 ⟌1650
    154
     110
     110
       0
```

Solution: 165 lb = 75 kg

SKILL SHARPENER

Convert the following from pounds to kilograms. Round to the nearest kilogram.

1. 220 lb ____________________

2. 175 lb ____________________

3. 40 lb ____________________

4. 12 lb ____________________

5. 195 lb ____________________

6. 155 lb ______________________

7. 90 lb ______________________

8. 120 lb ______________________

9. 200 lb ______________________

10. 6 lb ______________________

Convert the following from kilograms to pounds. Round to the nearest pound.

11. 55 kg ______________________

12. 100 kg ______________________

13. 110 kg ______________________

14. 22 kg ______________________

15. 12 kg ______________________

16. 90 kg ______________________

17. 155 kg ______________________

18. 80 kg ______________________

19. 125 kg ______________________

20. 130 kg ______________________

Objective

11.3 Read an English (household) ruler.

Health care providers should be able to accurately read and record length measurements using both English and metric measurements. The English ruler uses inches and fractions of inches, which may be combined to form feet and/or yards. An example of an English ruler is illustrated in Figure 11-2.

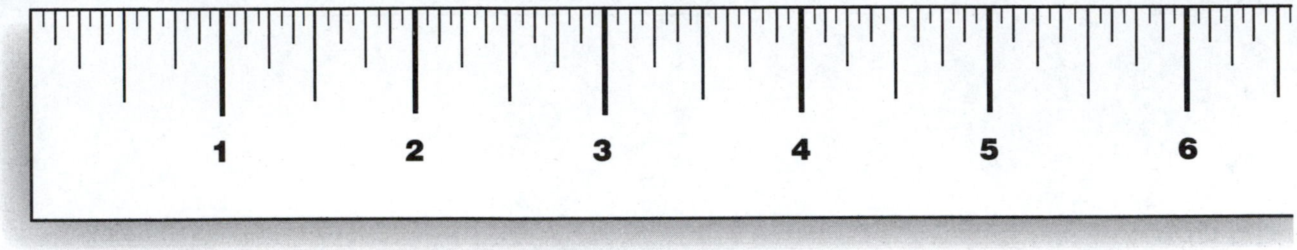

FIGURE 11-2 Household (English) ruler

To read the ruler, find the nearest inch mark to the left of the end of the item being measured. This is the number of inches. Then determine the fraction of an inch (if applicable) by determining where the end of the item being measured is. For example, this dropper measures 3 1/4 inches.

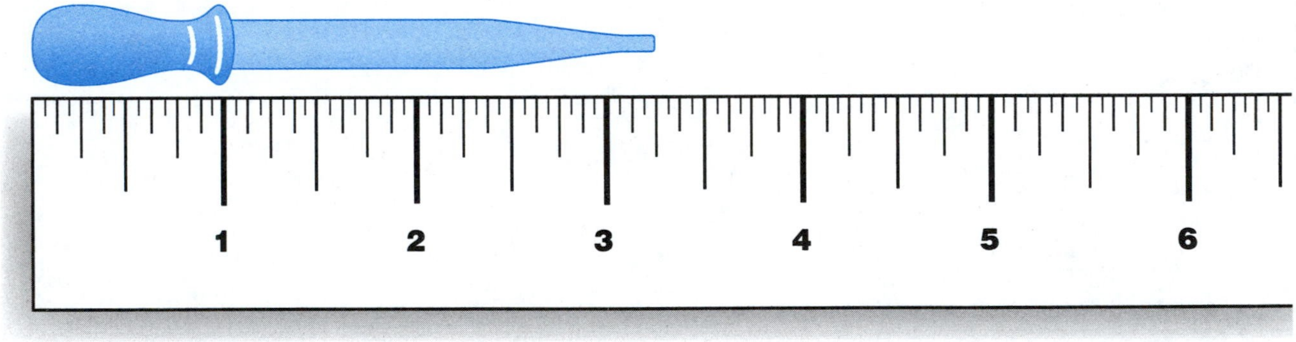

SKILL SHARPENER

Record the length of the following bars.

1. ______________________

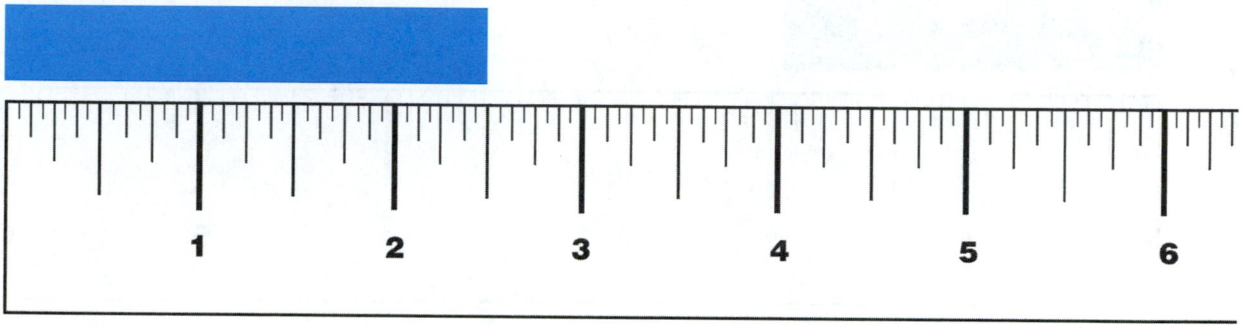

2. ______________________

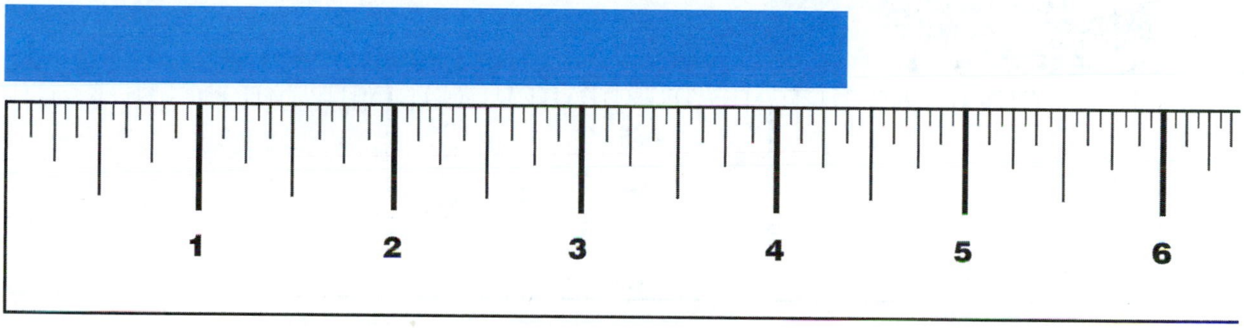

3. ______________________

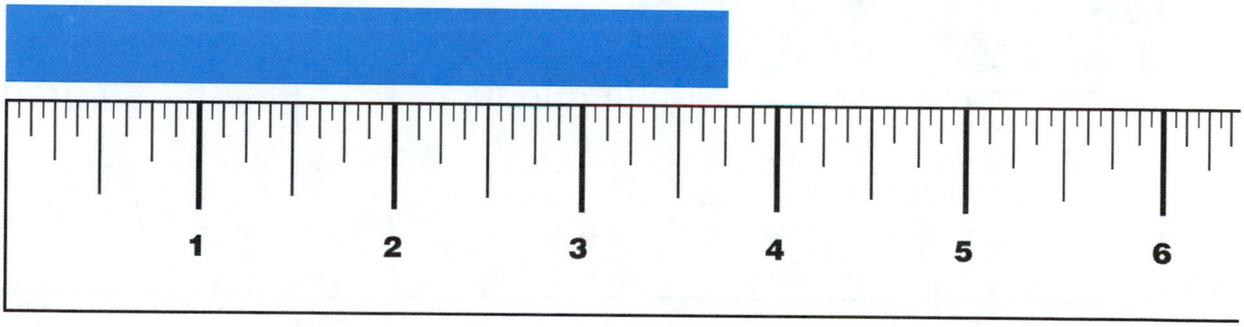

4. ________________________________

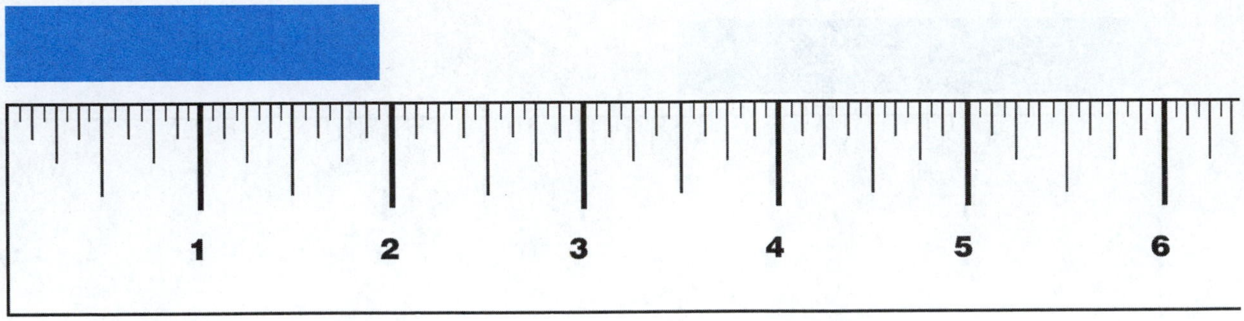

5. ________________________________

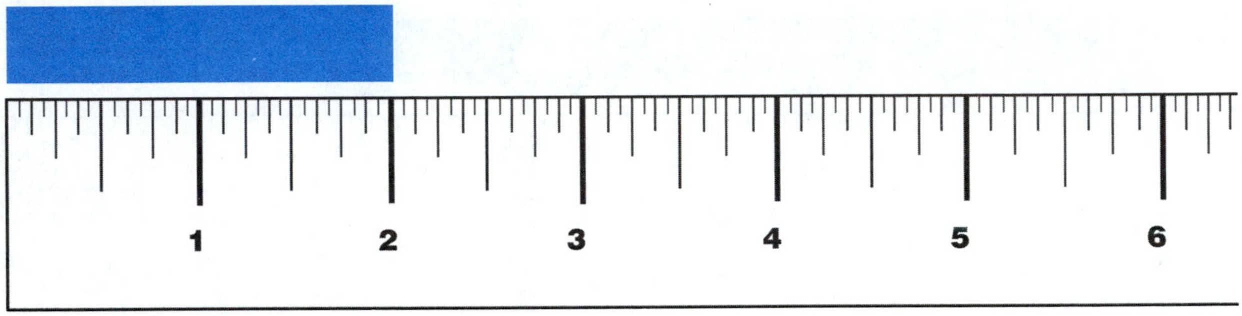

6. ________________________________

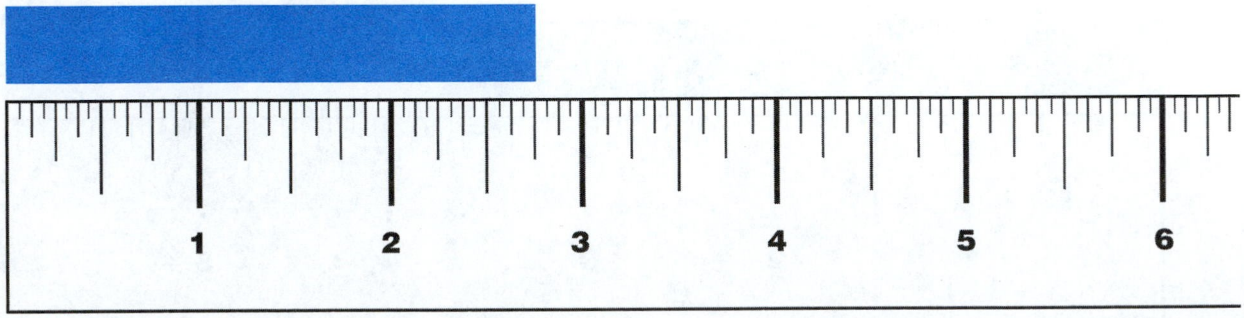

7. ______________________________

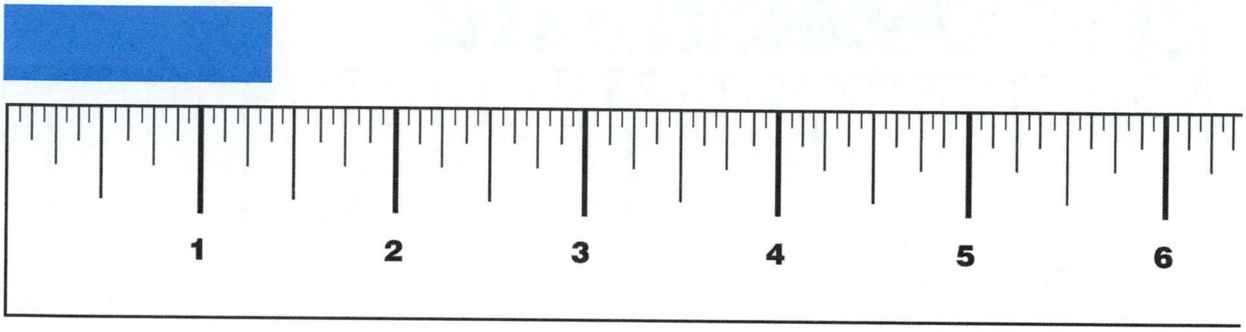

8. ______________________________

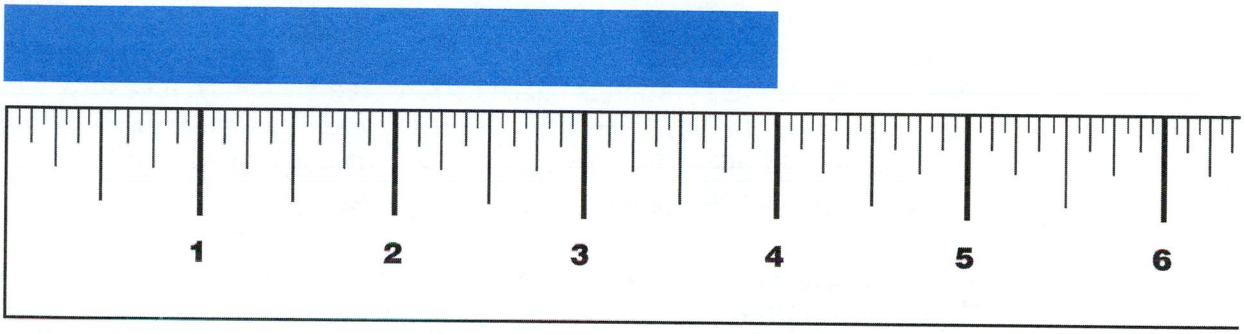

9. ______________________________

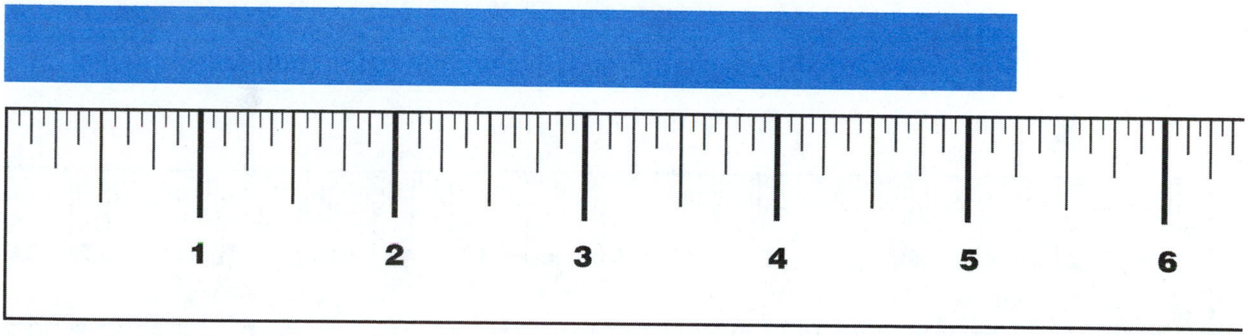

10. ______________________________

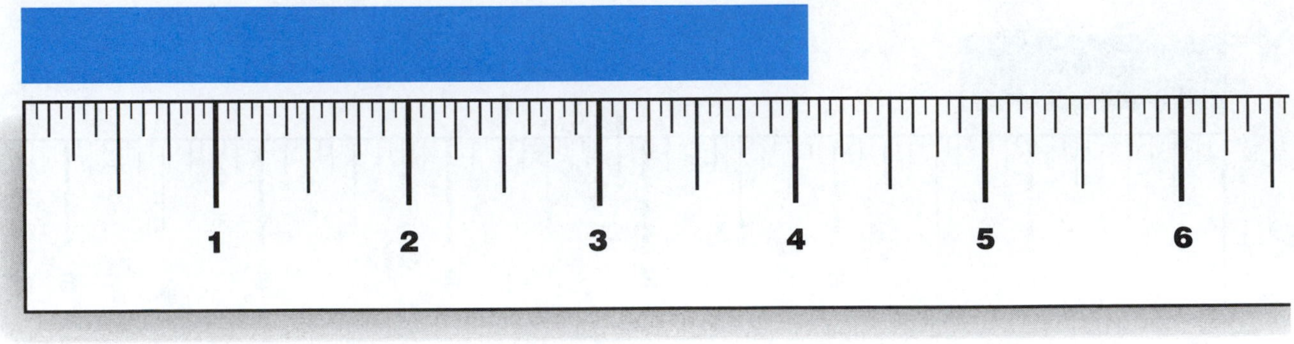

Objective

11.4 Read a metric ruler.

Because the metric system is based on tens, metric length measure is based on the meter. Lengths smaller than a meter are measured by tenths (decimeter), hundredths (centimeter), and thousandths (millimeter) of a meter, while lengths longer than a meter are measured by multiples of ten (decameter), hundreds (hectometer), and thousands (kilometer).

The metric ruler is based on centimeters and millimeters. To read the metric ruler, find the mark closest to the item you are measuring. If it is a longer mark noted by a number, measure by centimeters. If it is a shorter mark, use millimeters. For example, the ruler shown in Figure 11-3 shows a reading of 2 centimeters, or 20 millimeters.

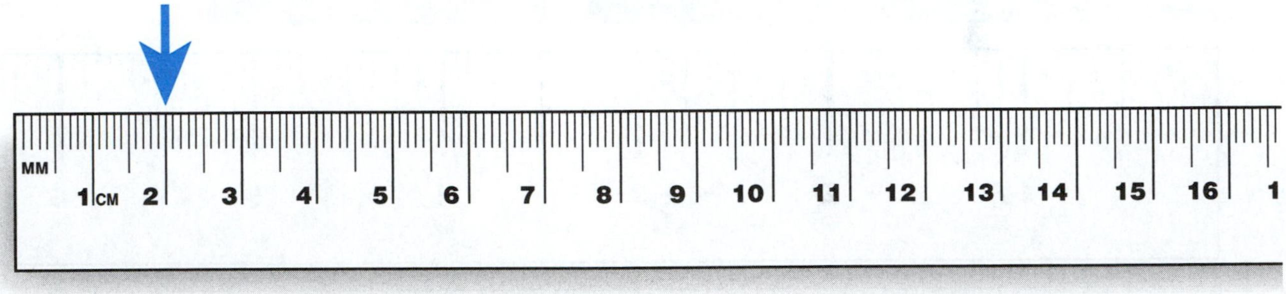

FIGURE 11-3 Metric ruler

SKILL SHARPENER

Note the lengths designated on each of the following rulers.

1. ______________________

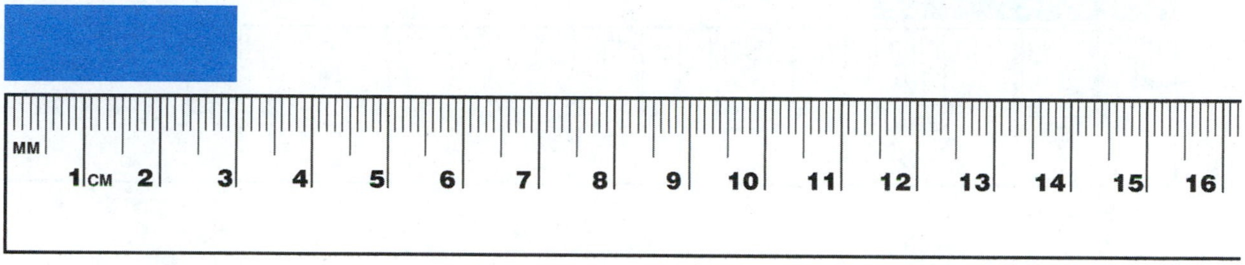

2. ______________________

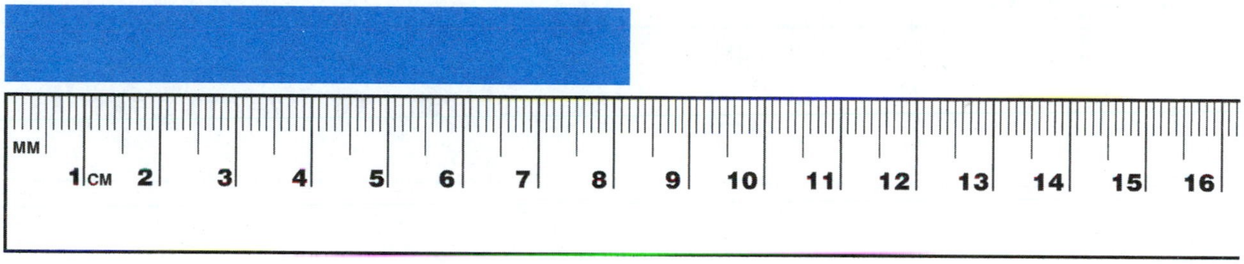

3. ______________________

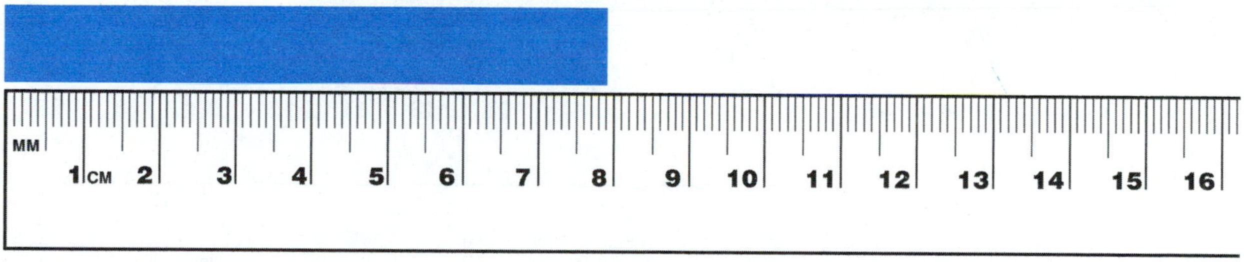

4. ______________________

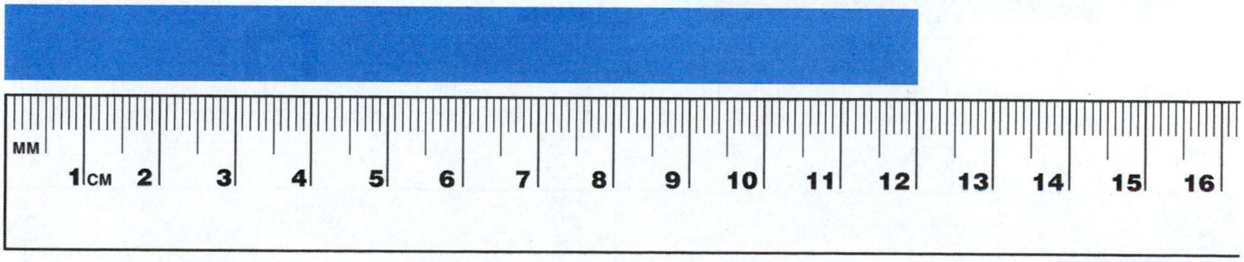

5. ______________________________

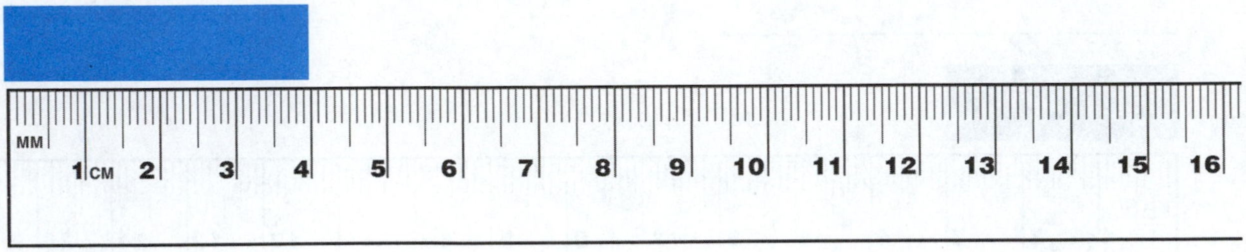
MM
1 CM 2 3 4 5 6 7 8 9 10 11 12 13 14 15 16

6. ______________________________

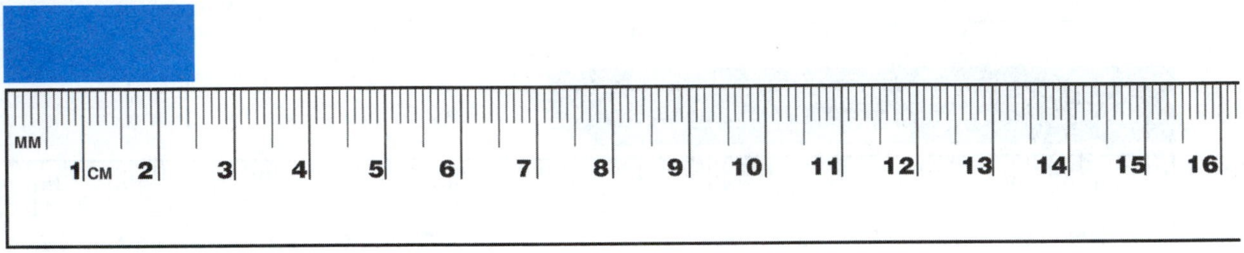
MM
1 CM 2 3 4 5 6 7 8 9 10 11 12 13 14 15 16

7. ______________________________

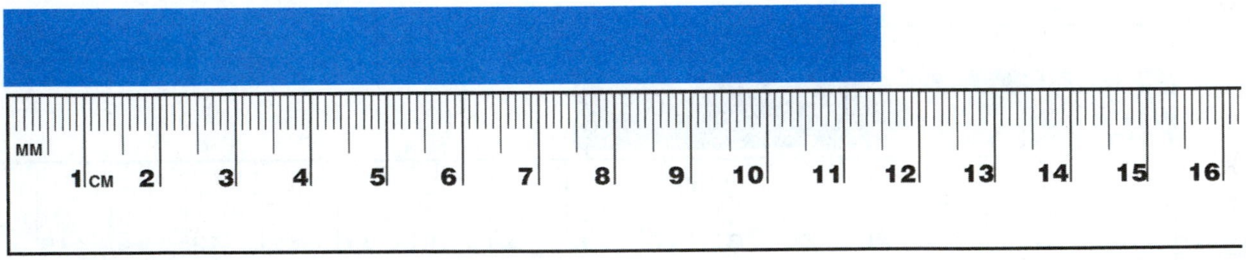
MM
1 CM 2 3 4 5 6 7 8 9 10 11 12 13 14 15 16

8. ______________________________

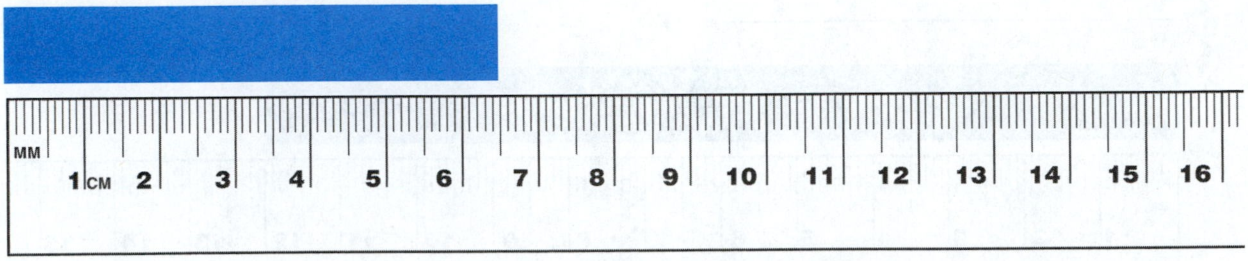
MM
1 CM 2 3 4 5 6 7 8 9 10 11 12 13 14 15 16

9. ____________________

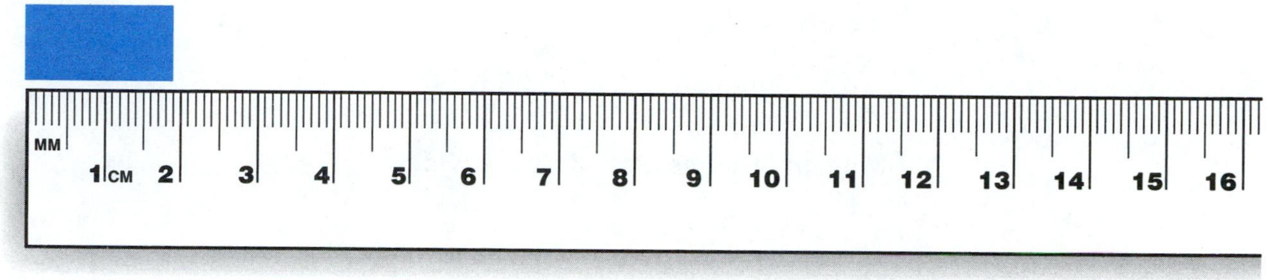

10. ____________________

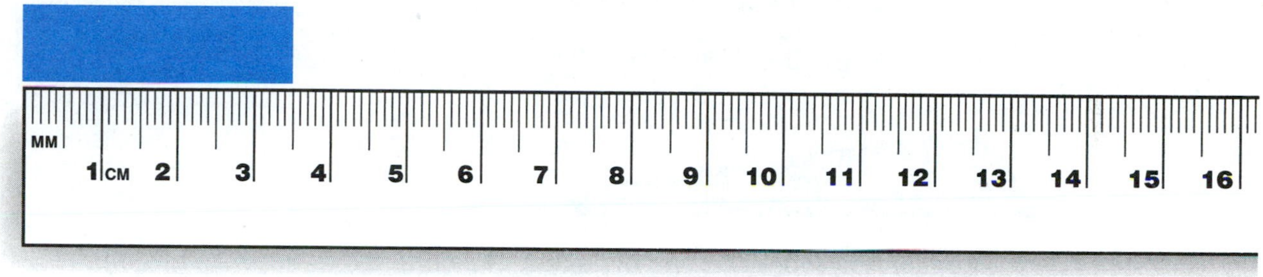

Objective

11.5 Convert between English and metric length measurements.

To convert between English and metric length measurements, you need to know the conversion factors or formulas. Key conversion formulas include the following.

1 inch	=	25.40 millimeters	= 2.54 centimeters	
1 foot	=	12 inches		
1 yard	=	3 feet		
1 meter	=	39.37 inches	= 3.28 feet	= 1.09 yards
1 dekameter	=	32.81 feet		
1 hectometer	=	328.08 feet		
1 kilometer	=	3280.08 feet	= 0.62 mile	
1 millimeter	=	0.04 inch		
1 centimeter	=	0.39 inch		
1 decimeter	=	3.94 inches		

Example: Convert 3 meters to feet.

The problem:

3 meters = _____ feet

Set up as:

3 m : x ft : : 1 m : 3.28 ft

Multiply the means. 3 : x :: 1 : 3.28

x × 1 = 1x or x

Multiply the extremes. 3 : x :: 1 : 3.28

3 × 3.28 = 9.84

Solution: x = 9.84

Therefore, 3 meters = 9.84 feet.

SKILL SHARPENER

Convert the following feet to meters. Round to the nearest hundredth.

1. 10 feet ____________________

2. 2 feet, 9 inches ____________________

3. 9 feet, 3 inches ____________________

4. 4 1/2 feet ____________________

5. 65 feet ____________________

6. 19 feet, 6 inches ______________________

7. 45 feet ______________________

8. 900 feet ______________________

9. 17.5 feet ______________________

10. 75 feet ______________________

Convert the following meters to feet.

11. 19 meters ______________________

12. 2.5 meters ______________________

13. 13 meters ______________________

14. 112 meters ______________________

15. 84 meters ____________________

16. 32 meters ____________________

17. 55 1/3 meters ____________________

18. 1 1/2 meters ____________________

19. 16 meters ____________________

20. 4 meters ____________________

Convert the following measurements to inches.

21. 3 feet ____________________

22. 2 feet ____________________

23. 2 1/2 feet ______________________

24. 5 feet, 3 inches ______________________

25. 1 1/2 meters ______________________

26. 2 meters ______________________

27. 3 1/3 feet ______________________

28. 2 feet, 4 inches ______________________

29. 1 foot, 9 inches ______________________

30. 4 meters ______________________

Objective

11.6 Read a thermometer.

Thermometers are instruments used to measure temperature. There are currently many types of thermometers available for use by health care professionals, including clinical glass thermometers, electronic thermometers, tympanic thermometers, and electronic thermometers. Figure 11-4 illustrates several types of thermometers.

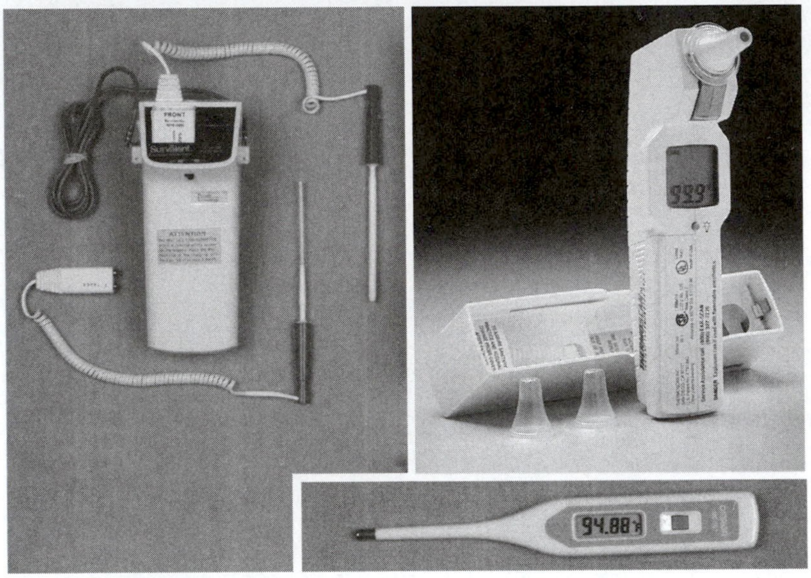

FIGURE 11-4 A variety of thermometers are available.

Most modern thermometers feature a digital readout, allowing the health care professional to simply read the temperature displayed in Hindu-Arabic numerals. Glass clinical thermometers, on the other hand, require some amount of skill and practice to secure an accurate reading. Figure 11-5 illustrates different types of glass clinical thermometers.

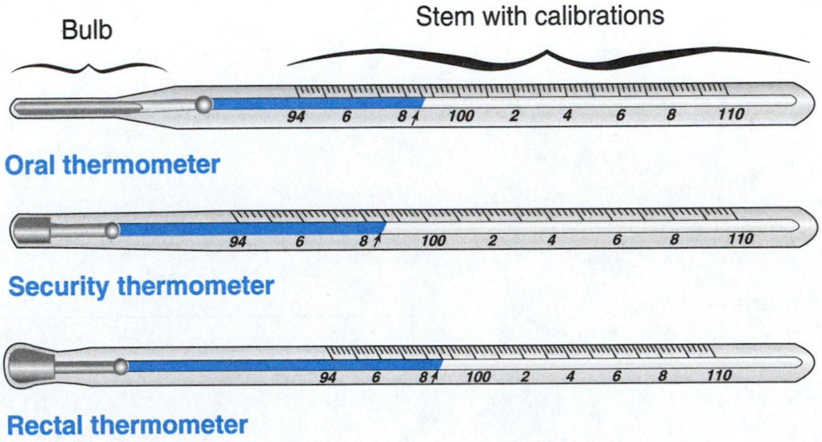

FIGURE 11-5 Types of clinical glass thermometers

Glass clinical thermometers are calibrated tubes that contain a column of colored liquid. Standard clinical thermometers start at 94°F with each long line indicating a one-degree elevation in temperature. Smaller lines indicate a 0.2°F variance in temperature. To read this type of thermometer, note the line at the end of the colored liquid and determine the number that the line represents. Figure 11-6 shows an example of how to read a clinical thermometer.

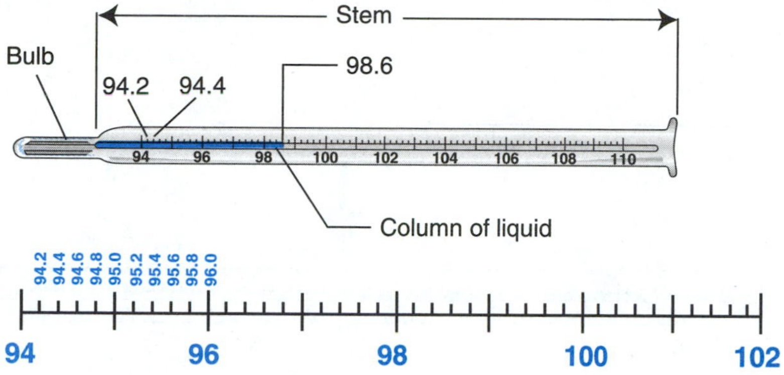

FIGURE 11-6 How to read a glass thermometer. This thermometer reads 98.6°F, the normal body core temperature.

SKILL SHARPENER

Identify the temperatures illustrated on each of the following thermometers.

1. ______________________________

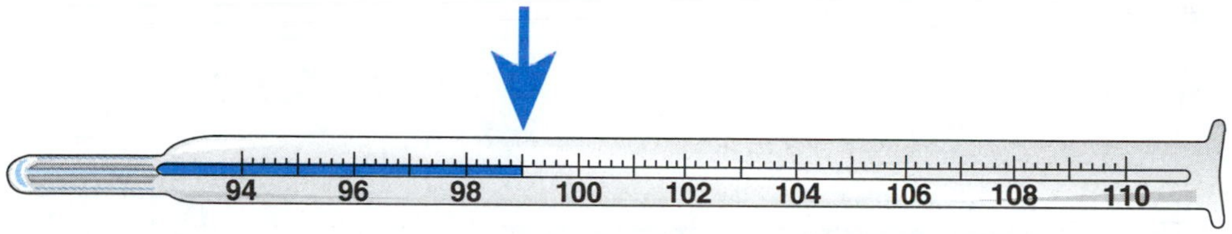

2. ______________________________

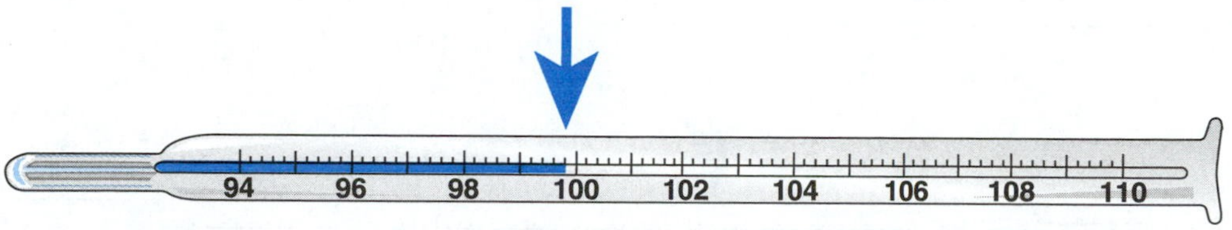

3. ______________________________

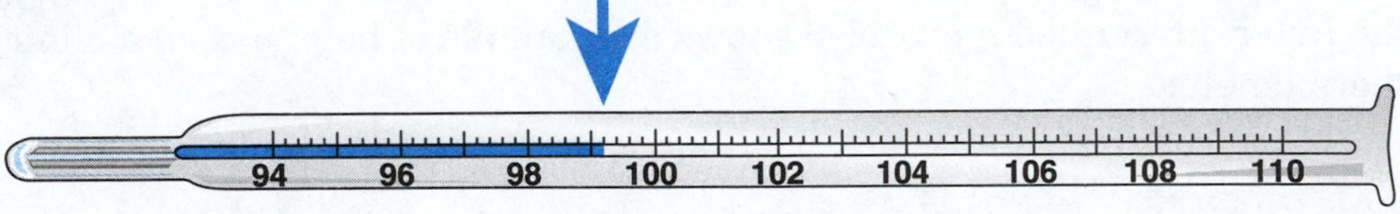
94
96
98
100
102
104
106
108
110

4. ______________________________

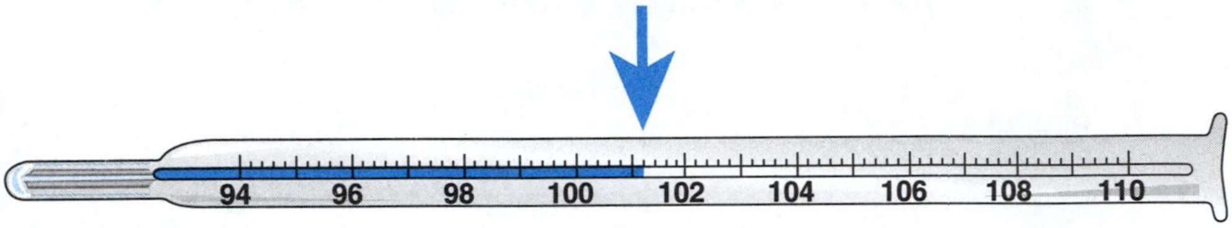
94
96
98
100
102
104
106
108
110

5. ______________________________

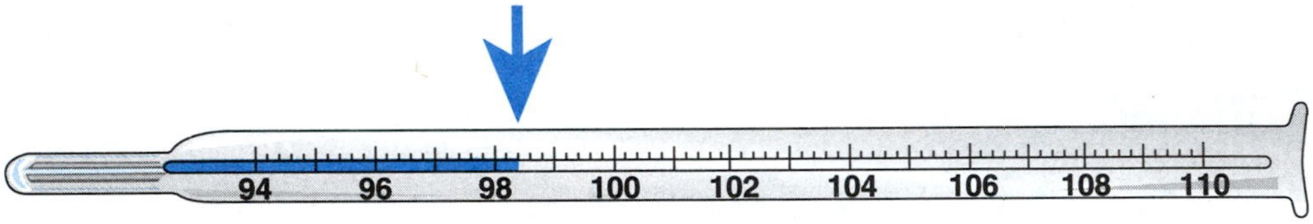
94
96
98
100
102
104
106
108
110

6. ______________________________

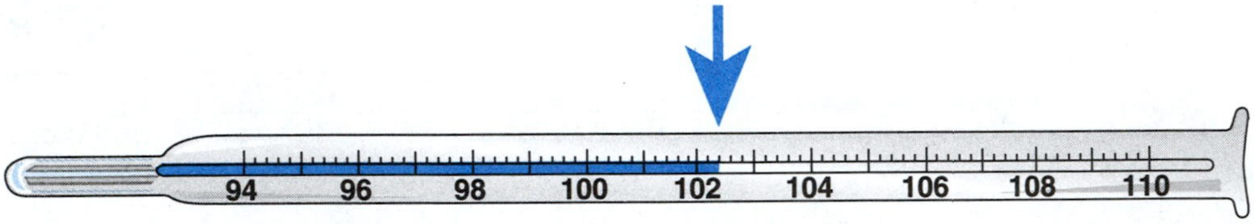
94
96
98
100
102
104
106
108
110

7. ______________________________

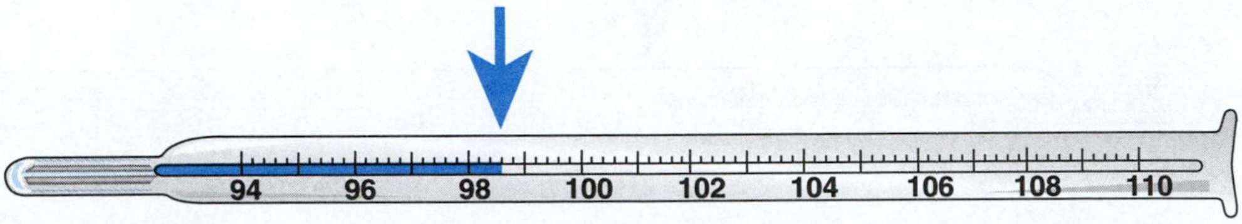
94
96
98
100
102
104
106
108
110

8. ____________________________

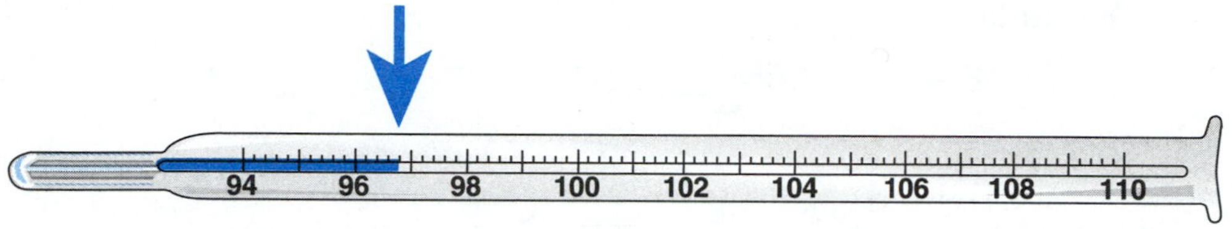

9. ____________________________

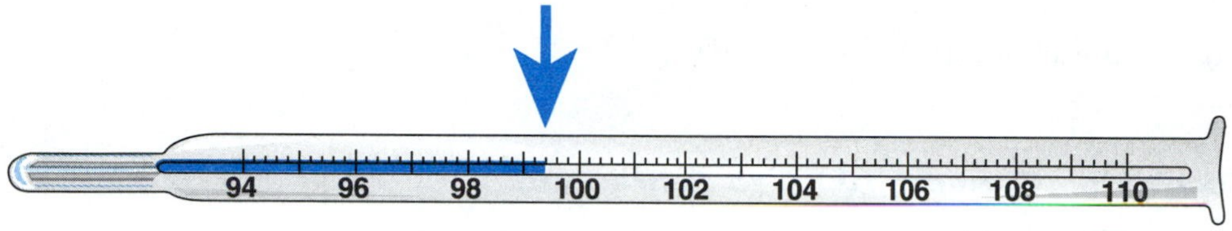

10. ____________________________

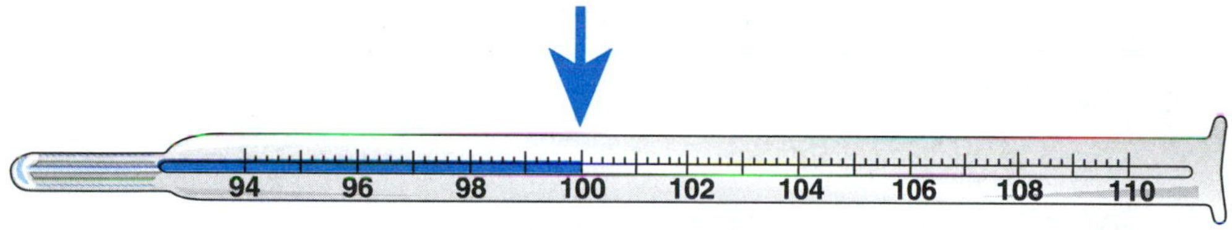

Objective

11.7 Convert between Fahrenheit and Celsius.

Fahrenheit is a thermometric scale in which water freezes at 32°F and boils at 212°F. **Celsius** is the international thermometric scale in which water freezes at 0°C and boils at 100°C. Sometimes it is necessary to convert between Fahrenheit (F) and Celsius (C) temperature measurements. To do this, use one of the following methods of conversion.

Fahrenheit to Celsius

$°F - 32 \div 1.8 = °C$

or

$°F - 32 \times \frac{5}{9} = °C$

Celsius to Fahrenheit

$°C \times 1.8 + 32 = °F$

or

$°C \times \frac{9}{5} + 32 = °F$

Example: Convert 100°F to Celsius.

The problem:

100°F = _____ °C

Formula:

°F − 32 ÷ 1.8 = _____ °C

Set up as:

100°F − 32 ÷ 1.8 = _____ °C

Solve.

(100 − 32) ÷ 1.8 = ______ °C

68 ÷ 1.8 = 37.77°C

Solution: 100°F = 37.77°C

Example: Convert 100°C to Fahrenheit.

The problem:

100°C = _____ °F

Formula:

°C × 1.8 + 32 = _____ °F

Set up as:

100°C × 1.8 + 32 = _____ °F

Solve.

(100 × 1.8) + 32 = ______ °F

180 + 32 = 212°F

Solution: 100°C = 212°F

SKILL SHARPENER

Convert from Fahrenheit to Celsius.

1. 120°F ______________________

2. 41°F ______________________

3. 99.6°F ______________________

4. 101.3°F ______________________

5. 102.9°F ______________________

6. 200°F ______________________

7. 90°F ______________________

8. 104.5°F ______________________

9. 110°F ______________________

10. 55°F ______________________

Convert from Celsius to Fahrenheit.

11. 32°C ____________

12. 87°C ____________

13. 12.9°C ____________

14. 43°C ____________

15. 55°C ____________

16. 76°C ____________

17. 22.9°C ____________

18. 35°C ______________________

19. 16.8°C ______________________

20. 75°C ______________________

Objective

11.8 Determine body surface area.

Body surface area (BSA) is used to determine drug dosages for infants and children, as well as a select group of adult patients. A mathematical estimate, expressed in square meters (m^2) of body surface area, is calculated based on the height and weight of the patient. Body surface area may be estimated through a mathematical calculation or by using a **nomogram**, a graphic image in which a straight line connects known values to find an unknown value. A nomogram for estimating body surface area is illustrated in Figure 11-7.

To use the nomogram, first determine the height and weight of the patient. Place a straight edge extending from the patient's weight in the right column to the patient's height in the left column. Now look at the place where the straight edge intersects the surface area (SA) column. This is the patient's estimated body surface area. If the patient is a child with normal height for his or her weight, the second column from the left (as illustrated in Figure 11-8) should be used.

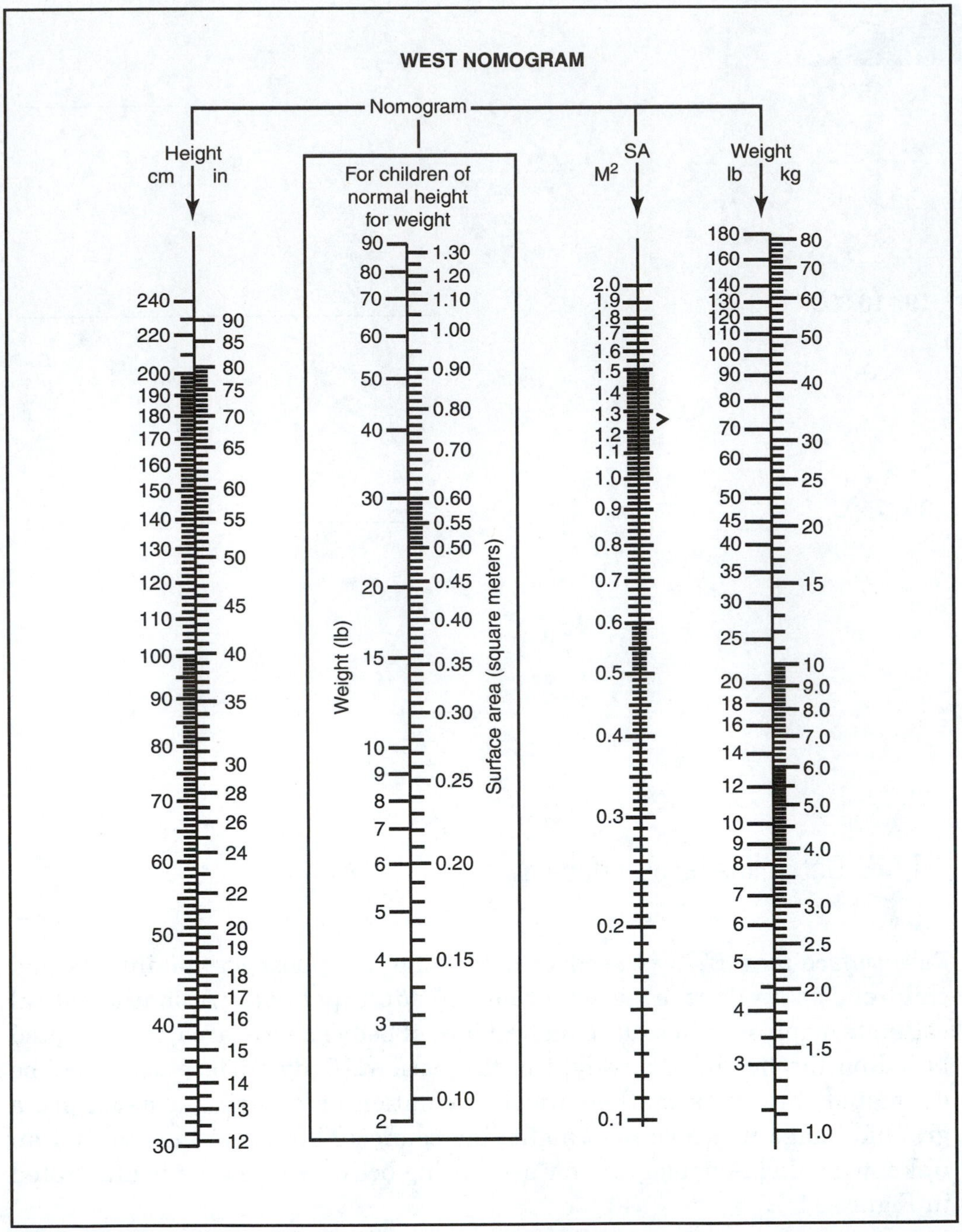

FIGURE 11-7 This nomogram may be used to estimate body surface area (BSA).

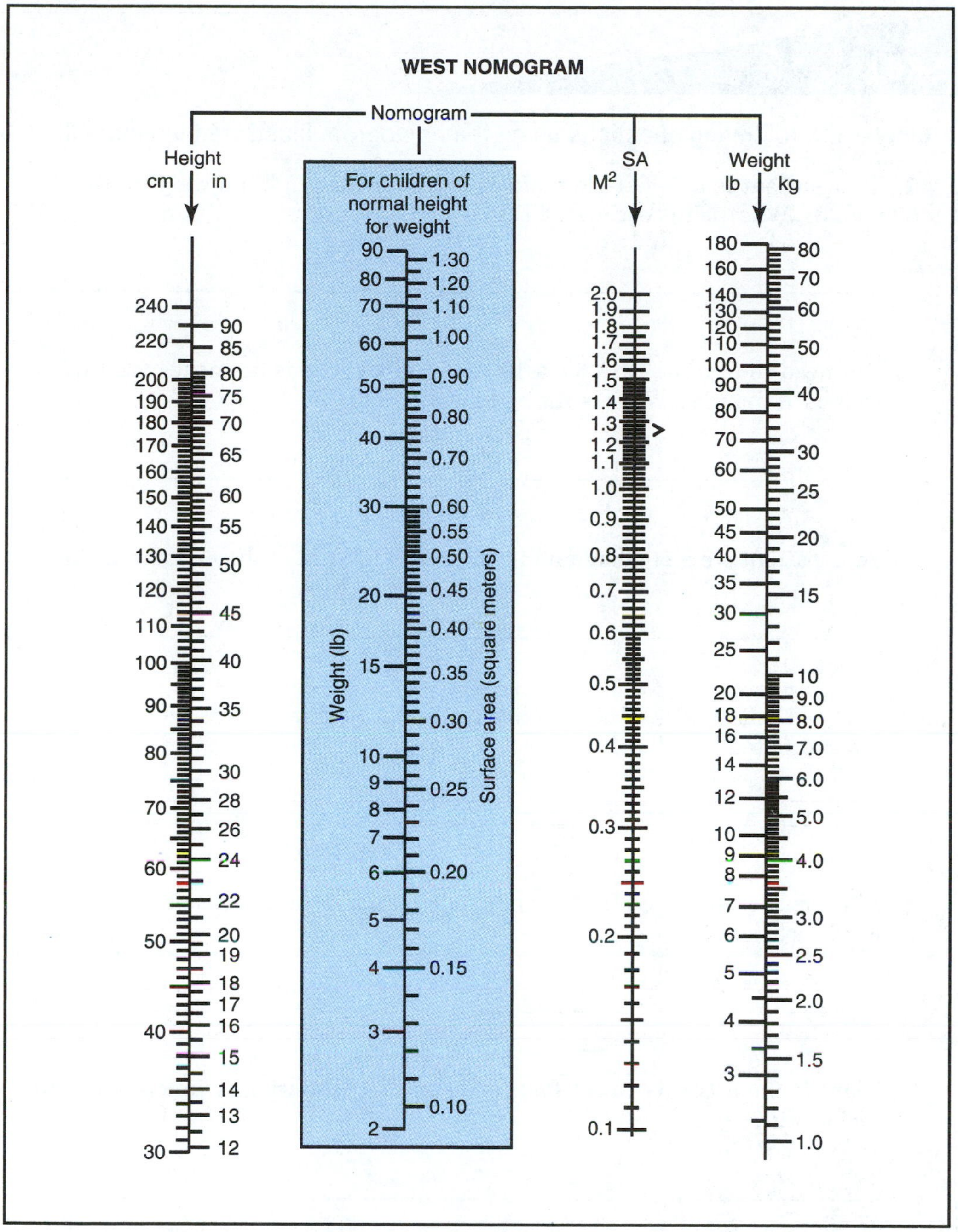

FIGURE 11-8 This nomogram may be used for children of normal height for their weight.

SKILL SHARPENER

Answer the following questions using the nomogram illustrated in Figure 11-7.

1. Your patient is a 7-year-old male who is 50 inches tall and weighs 50 pounds. What is his estimated BSA?

____

2. You need to find the BSA for a 10-year-old boy who is 55 inches tall and weighs 70 pounds. What is his estimated BSA?

____

3. Your patient weighs 40 kg and is 150 cm tall. What is the estimated BSA?

____

4. Your patient, who is of normal height for his weight, weighs 30 lb. What is his estimated BSA?

____

5. What is the estimated BSA for a female patient who weighs 65 pounds and is 60 inches tall?

____

6. What is the estimated BSA for a male patient who weighs 75 kg and is 70 inches tall?

____

7. What is the estimated BSA for a patient who is 190 cm and 60 kg?

____

8. Determine the BSA for a patient who weighs 30 lb and is of normal height for her weight.

____

9. What is the estimated BSA for a 10-lb infant?

____

10. What is the estimated BSA for a patient of normal height for his weight of 25 lb?

____

CONCLUSION

The ability of a health care provider to accurately read and document weights, lengths, and temperatures is vital to providing quality patient care. Accuracy is important, since weights and measurements affect medication dosages, and temperature is an important vital sign that may provide valuable insight into the patient's condition.

REVIEW AND REFLECT

1. Describe a situation in which a health care professional might need to convert between the English and metric systems of measure.

____

____

____

____

____

2. Which measurement provides more accuracy: kilograms or pounds? Why?

____

____

____

____

____

3. With which measurement system do you feel more comfortable? Why?

4. Explain advantages of using the metric system.

5. Explain advantages of using the English system.

CHAPTER 12

Measuring Intake and Output

LEARNING OBJECTIVES

After completing this chapter, the reader will be able to:

- **12.1** Define intake and output.
- **12.2** Accurately measure urinary output.
- **12.3** Determine total daily output.
- **12.4** Determine intake by estimating.
- **12.5** Discover fluid imbalances by comparing intake and output.

KEY TERMS

- dehydration
- intake
- output
- overhydration

MATH IN THE REAL WORLD

"Most clinicians do not understand the importance of accurately measuring intake and output..."

Mike Harper, CRNA, JD

SELF-ASSESSMENT **PRETEST**

Determine the amount of fluid in each of the following containers.

1. ______________________________

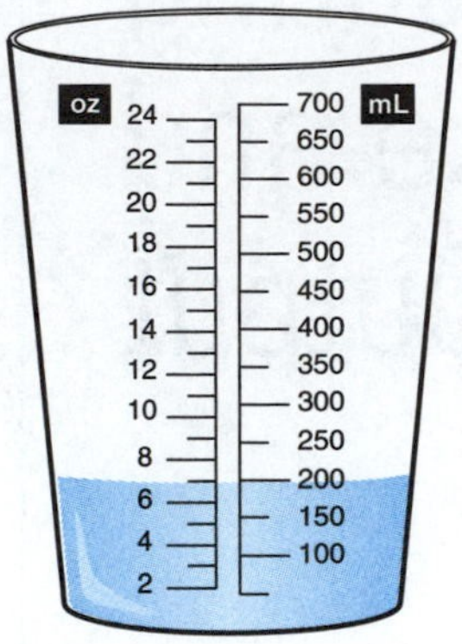

2. ______________________________

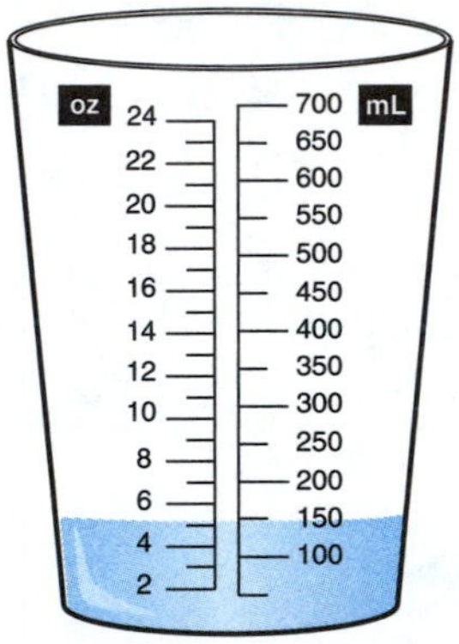

3. ______________________________

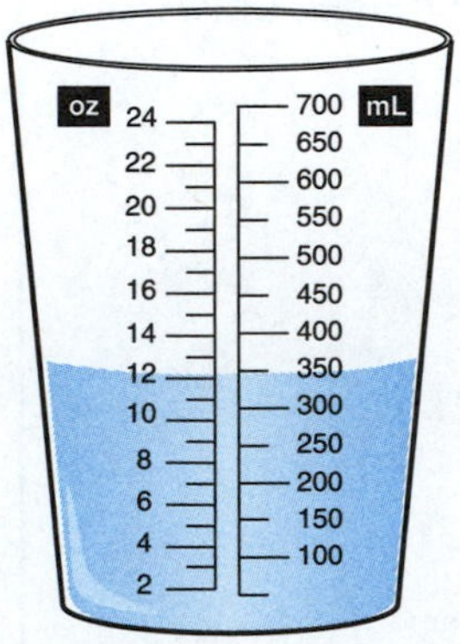

4. ______________________________

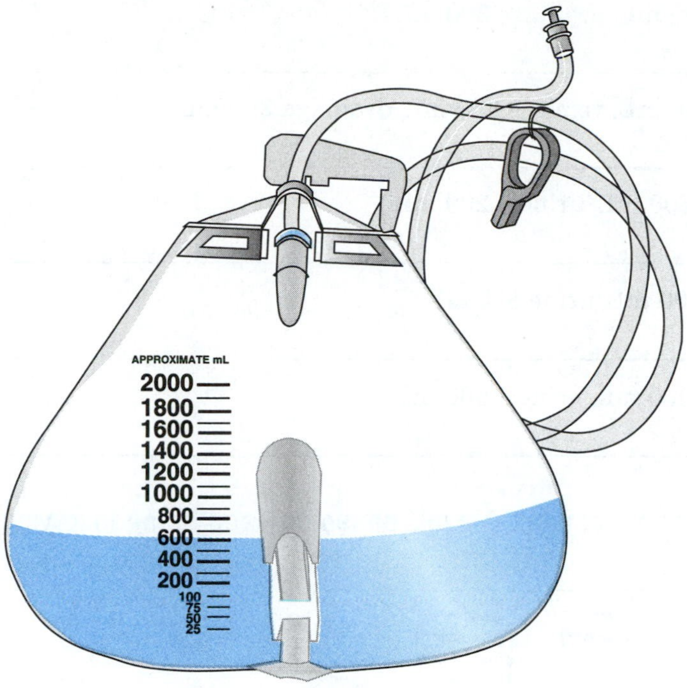
APPROXIMATE mL
2000
1800
1600
1400
1200
1000
800
600
400
200
100
75
50
25

5. ______________________________

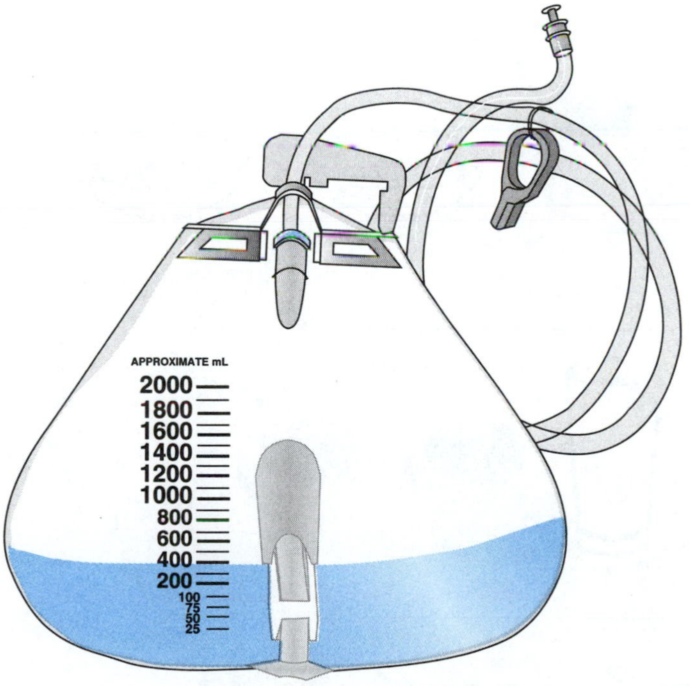
APPROXIMATE mL
2000
1800
1600
1400
1200
1000
800
600
400
200
100
75
50
25

Find the total daily output in each of the following.

6. urine 1,800 mL, drainage 300 mL

____

7. urine 2,000 mL, vomitus 350 mL, drainage 200 mL

____

8. drainage 600 mL, urine 1,200 mL

____

9. vomitus 800 mL, urine 850 mL

____

10. drainage 500 mL, urine 1,900 mL

____

Estimate the amount of intake, in mL, based on each of the following.

11. ______________________________

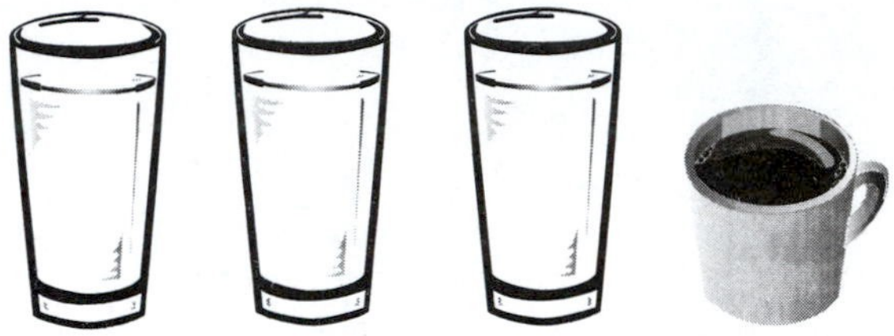

12. ______________________________

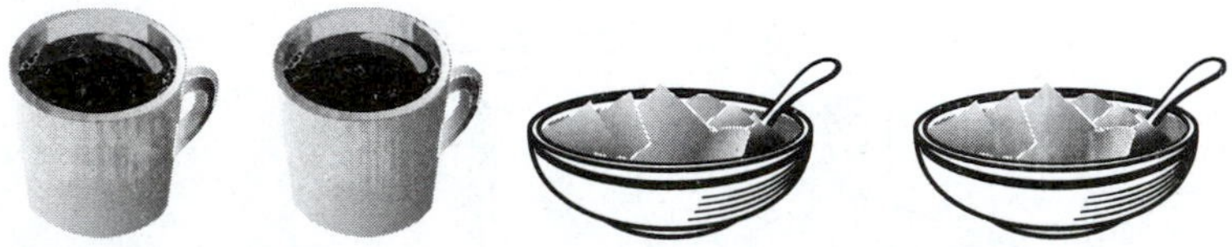

13. ______________________________

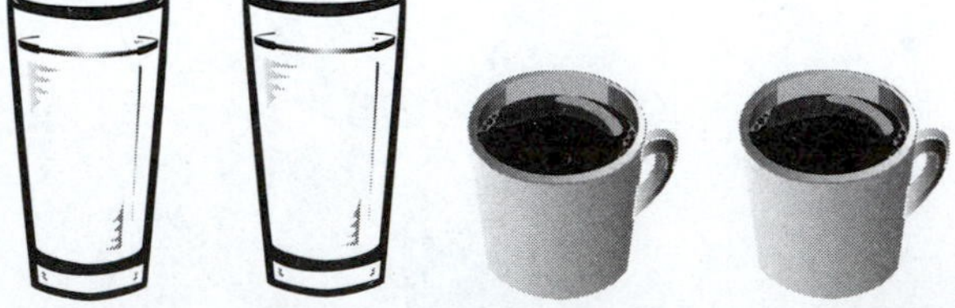

14. ______________________________

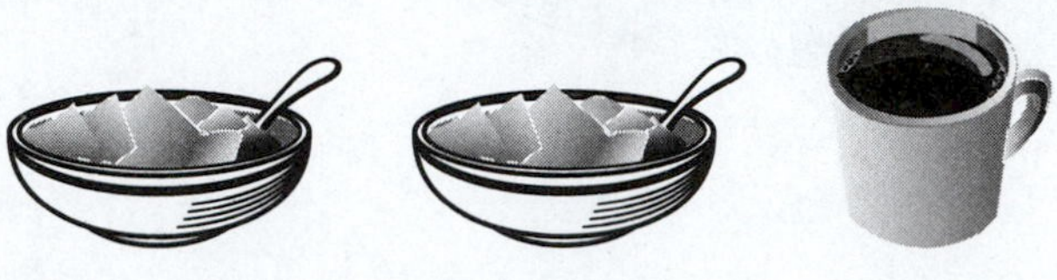

15. ______________________________

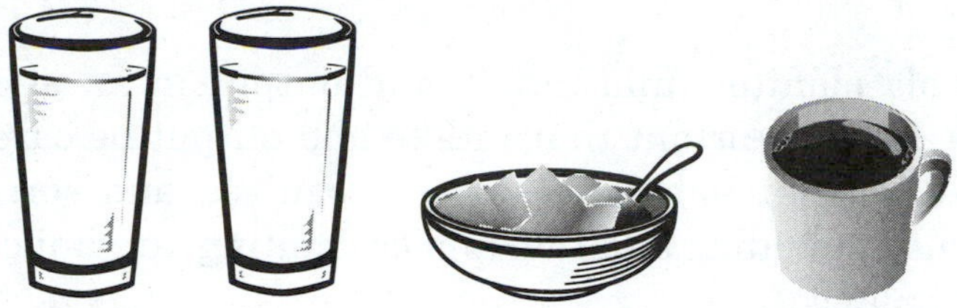

16. 1 glass of water ______________________________

17. 2 cups of coffee ______________________________

18. 1/2 serving of gelatin ______________________________

19. 2/3 glass of milk ______________________________

20. 1/2 bowl of soup ______________________________

Determine the balance between intake and output.

21. A patient had a total intake of 2,000 mL yesterday. Output included 1,500 mL of urine and 400 mL of fluid from drainage.

____

22. Your patient had a total daily output of 1,800 mL. According to her intake chart, she drank 6 glasses of water, 1/2 cup of coffee, 2 glasses of tea, and 2 servings of gelatin.

____

23. The resident in an extended care facility had a total intake of 2,200 mL and output of 2,000 mL urine and 250 mL vomitus.

____

24. A patient had a daily output of 2,500 mL. According to records, he drank 2 glasses of water, 3 cups of coffee, 4 glasses of tea, and 1 1/2 servings of gelatin.

____

25. The patient had a daily intake of 1,900 mL and an urinary output as follows: 150 mL, 250 mL, 200 mL, 200 mL, 350 mL, 150 mL, 350 mL, and 200 mL.

____

INTRODUCTION

Health care professionals monitor fluid intake and output in an effort to maintain fluid balance. It is important that intake and output be carefully measured and recorded so that imbalances are recognized and corrected early. Mathematical skills, including addition and estimating, are important in monitoring for fluid balance.

Objective

12.1 Define intake and output.

Intake refers to anything that goes into the body, either by mouth or intravenously. **Output** refers to liquid that is removed from the body. It is important that intake and output be balanced to prevent **dehydration**, or fluid deficit, and **overhydration**, or fluid excess.

Objective

12.2 Accurately measure urinary output.

Under several circumstances, urinary output should be measured to help determine the balance between intake and output. Often, health care professionals must measure urine in a graduated container or in a urinary catheter drainage bag. It is important that these measurements be taken and recorded accurately so that health care professionals recognize fluid imbalances and prescribe appropriate actions should imbalances occur.

To measure urinary output in a graduated container (Figure 12-1), place the container on a level surface and read the measurement at the nearest line.

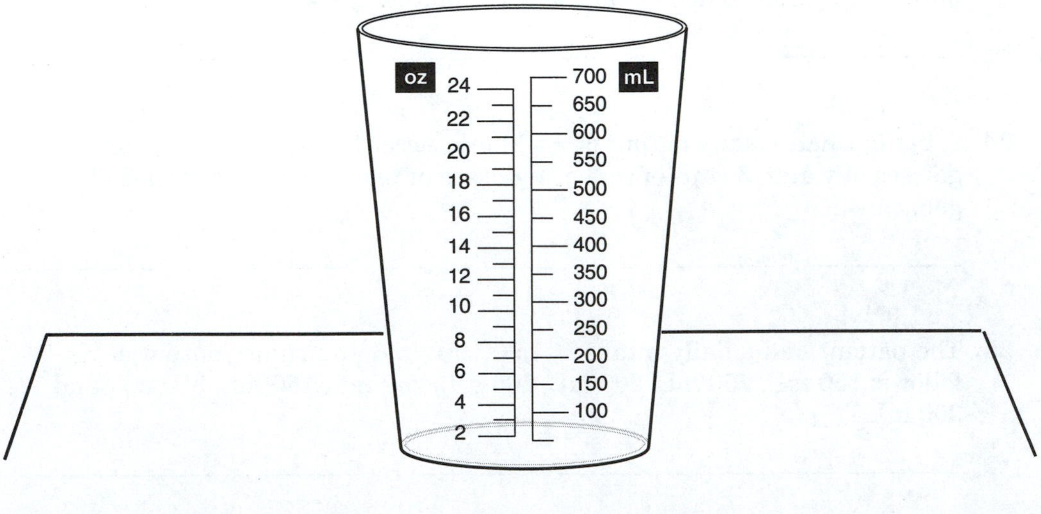

FIGURE 12-1 Place the graduated container on a flat surface for an accurate reading.

To measure urinary output in a urinary bag (Figure 12-2), read the container at the nearest line.

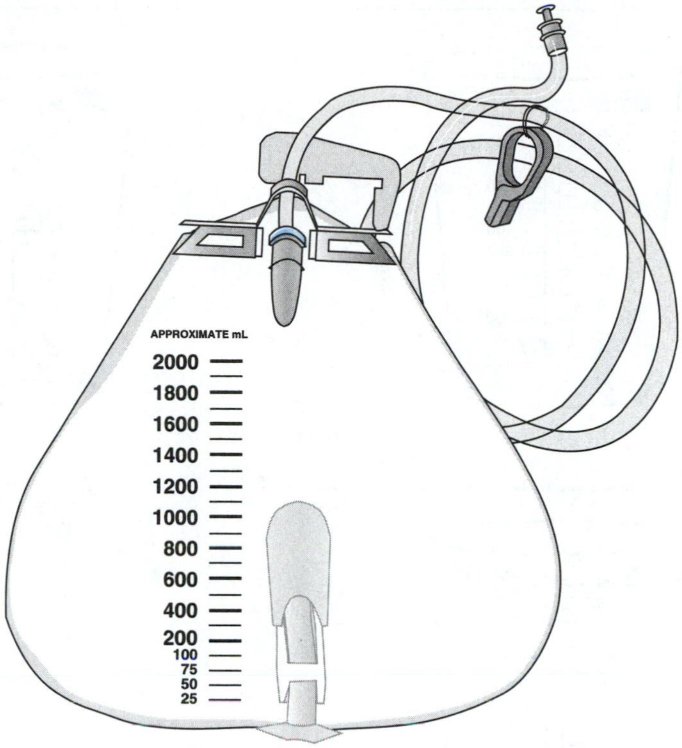

FIGURE 12-2 Urinary bags should be read level.

SKILL SHARPENER

Determine the total urinary output for each container.

1. ______________________

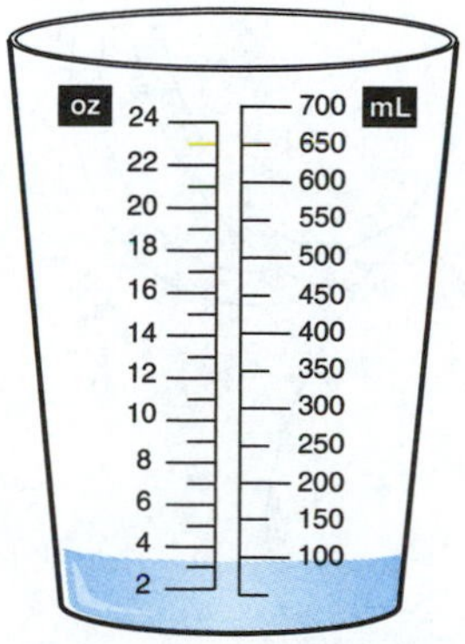

2. ______________________

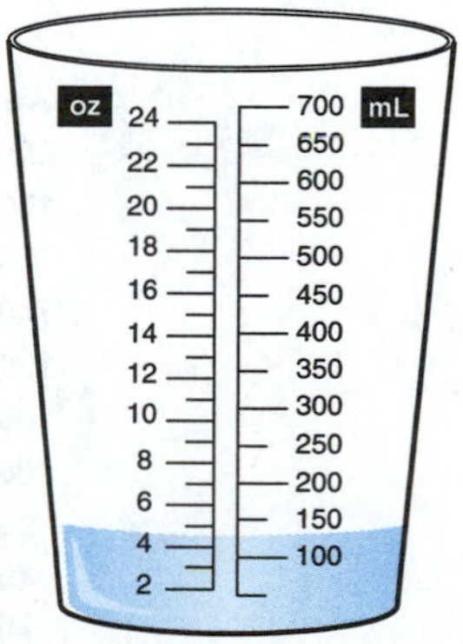

3. ______________________

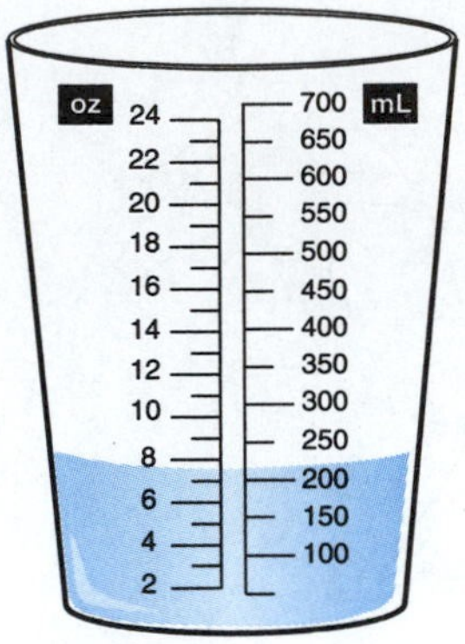
oz
24
22
20
18
16
14
12
10
8
6
4
2
700
650
600
550
500
450
400
350
300
250
200
150
100
mL

4. ______________________

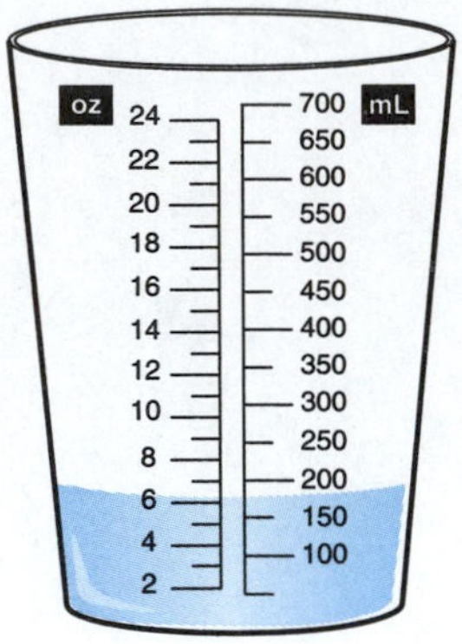
oz
24
22
20
18
16
14
12
10
8
6
4
2
700
650
600
550
500
450
400
350
300
250
200
150
100
mL

5. ______________________

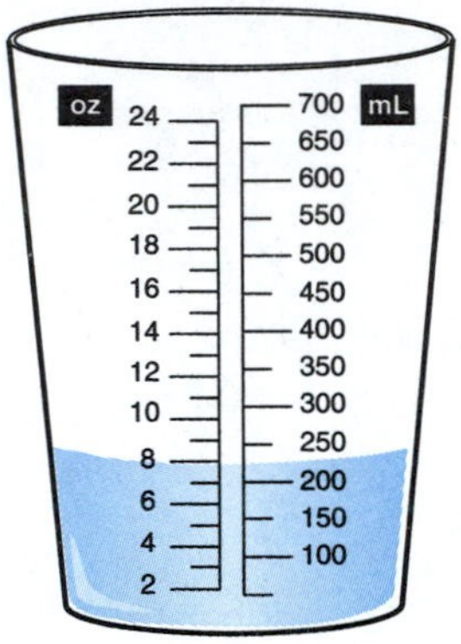
oz
24
22
20
18
16
14
12
10
8
6
4
2
700
650
600
550
500
450
400
350
300
250
200
150
100
mL

6. ______________________

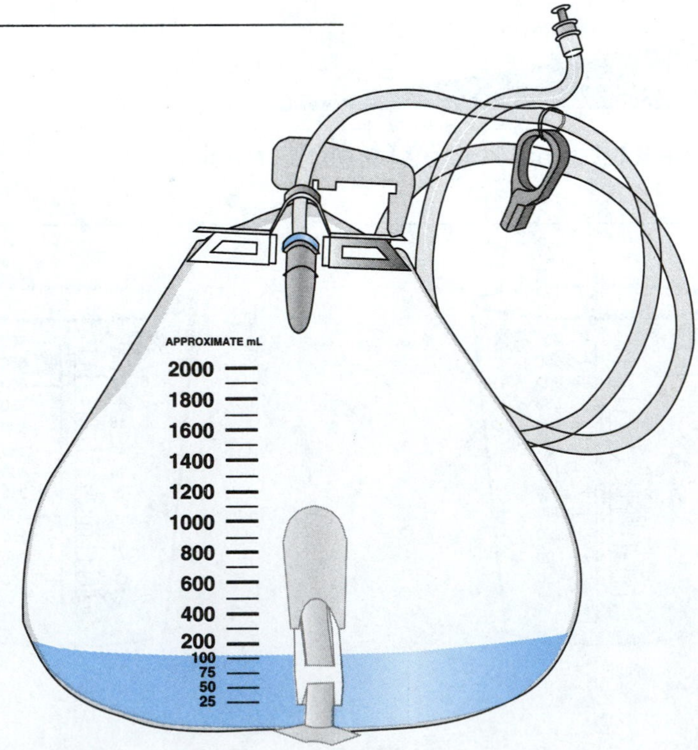
APPROXIMATE mL
2000
1800
1600
1400
1200
1000
800
600
400
200
100
75
50
25

7. ______________________________

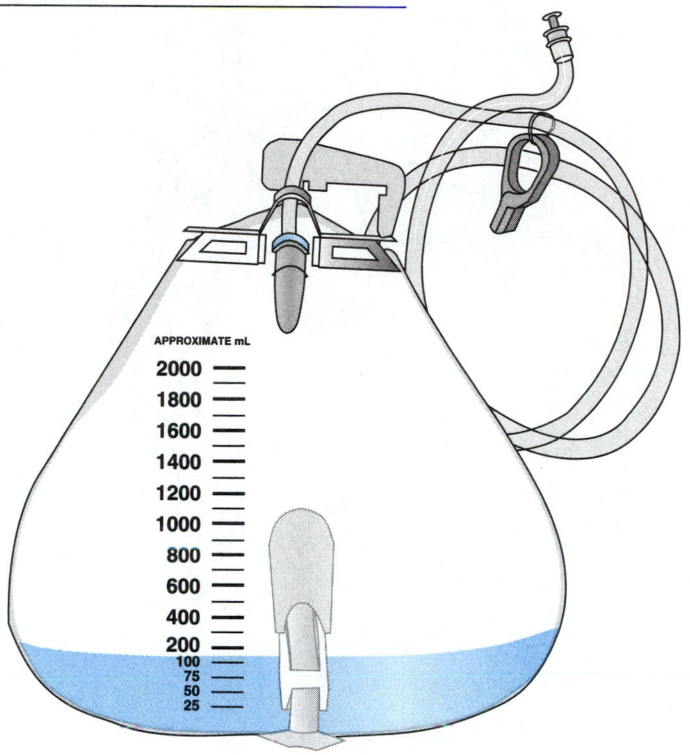
APPROXIMATE mL
2000
1800
1600
1400
1200
1000
800
600
400
200
100
75
50
25

8. ______________________________

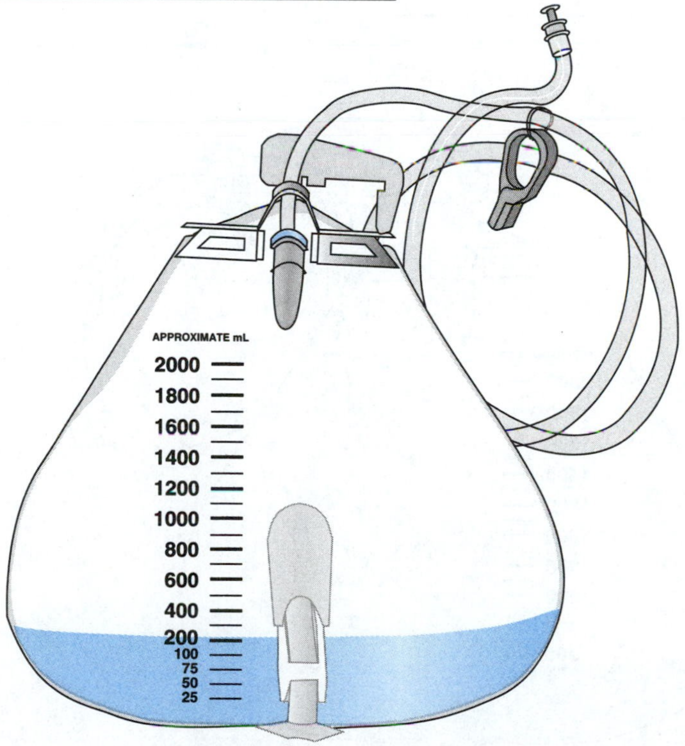
APPROXIMATE mL
2000
1800
1600
1400
1200
1000
800
600
400
200
100
75
50
25

9. ______________________________

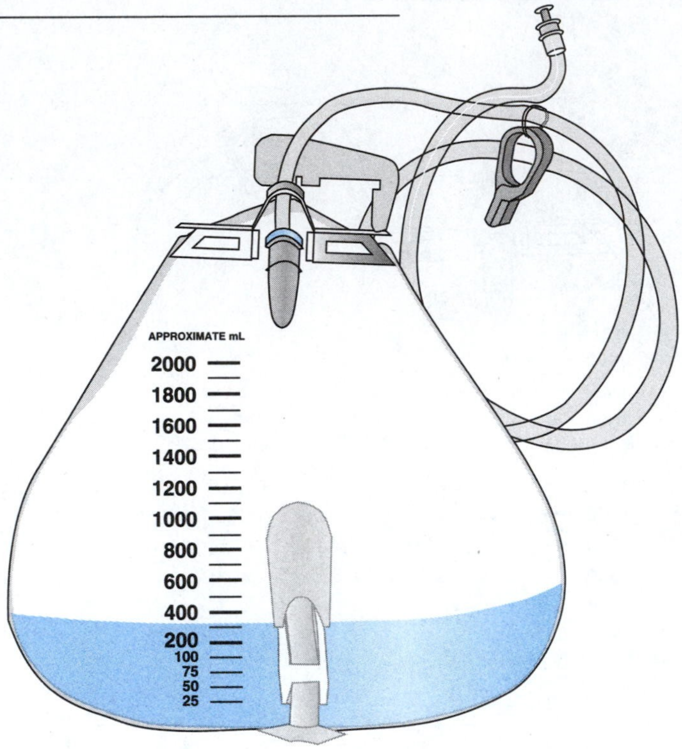
APPROXIMATE mL
2000
1800
1600
1400
1200
1000
800
600
400
200
100
75
50
25

10. ______________________________

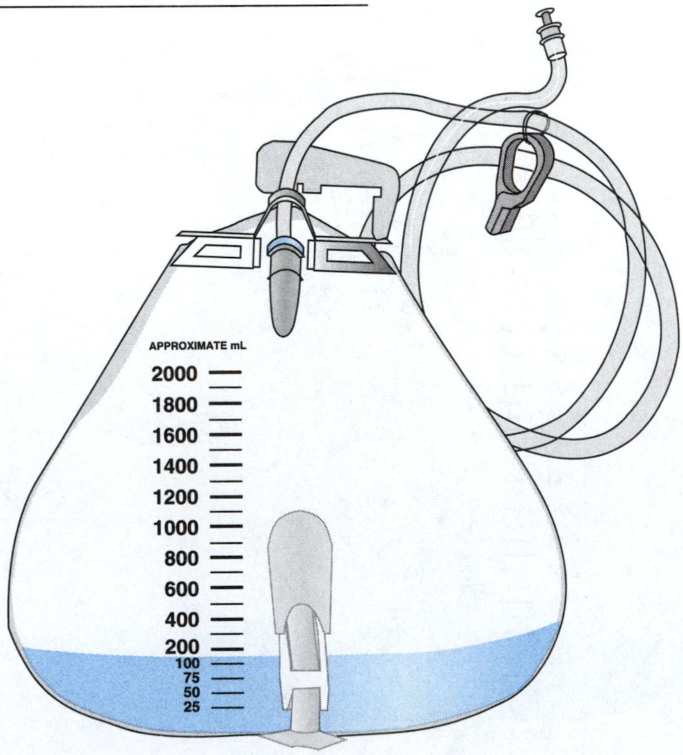
APPROXIMATE mL
2000
1800
1600
1400
1200
1000
800
600
400
200
100
75
50
25

Objective

12.3 Determine total daily output.

The total daily output is the amount of fluid excreted from the body during a 24-hour period. Normally, this total daily output should be approximately the same as the total daily intake and should be in the range of approximately 1,500–2,000 mL.

SKILL SHARPENER

Add the following recordings of output to determine the total daily output.

1. 1,000 mL of urine, 300 mL of vomitus, and 500 mL of drainage

____

2. 1,500 mL of urine, 200 mL of drainage

____

3. 2,000 mL of urine, 120 mL of vomitus

____

4. 1,900 mL of urine, 200 mL of drainage, and 300 mL of vomitus

____

5. Urine outputs of 350, 300, 250, 250, 350, and 250 mL

____

6. Urine outputs of 400, 350, 400, 345, 255, and 400 mL and 300 mL of vomitus

____

7. Urine outputs of 300, 200, 225, 175, 300, 245, and 300 mL and 400 mL of drainage

____

8. Drainage of 200 mL and urinary output totaling 1,900 mL

____

9. Vomitus totaling 400 mL and urinary output totaling 1,300 mL

____

10. 2,000 mL of urine, 100 mL of drainage, and 200 mL of vomitus

____

Objective

12.4 Determine intake by estimating.

Since the health care professional may need an estimate of input to determine fluid balance, it is helpful to be able to estimate intake based on serving sizes and the amount the patient has eaten. To make this task easier, several estimation guides similar to the following exist.

Coffee/tea cup	8 oz = 240 mL
Glass	8 oz = 240 mL
Water carafe	16 oz = 480 mL
Foam cup	8 oz = 240 mL
Soup bowl	6 oz = 180 mL
Gelatin	1 serving = 130 mL
Ice chips	4 oz glass = 120 mL

SKILL SHARPENER

Estimate the amount of intake based on the following.

1. one glass of milk and 1/2 cup of coffee

____

2. 1 cup of gelatin and 1/2 glass of orange juice

____

3. 2 cups of gelatin, 2 cups of coffee, and 1/2 glass of tea

____

4. 8 glasses of water, 3 glasses of milk, and 3 servings of gelatin

____

5. 1/2 cup of coffee, 1/2 glass of juice, 4 glasses of tea, and 2 glasses of water

____

Objective

12.5 Discover fluid imbalances by comparing intake and output.

By comparing total daily intake and total daily output, the health care provider determines if fluid imbalances exist. Early recognition of imbalances helps to prevent dehydration or overhydration of the hospitalized or institutionalized patient.

SKILL SHARPENER

Determine the fluid balance or imbalance of the following patients.

1. Mr. Genheim had a total fluid intake of 1,900 mL and a total fluid output of 1,850 mL.

   ____

2. Mrs. Reed drank six glasses of water and ate four servings of gelatin. Her output includes urine output of 250 mL, 200 mL, 300 mL, 275 mL, 200 mL, and 295 mL.

   ____

3. Mrs. Ahsirt had a total fluid intake of 2,000 mL and a total fluid output of 2,000 mL.

   ____

4. Mr. Jones drank 6 glasses of water, 3 glasses of juice, 2 cups of coffee, 2 cups of soup, and 3 servings of gelatin. What should his output be to achieve fluid balance?

   ____

5. Ms. Benjamin ate 3 cups of soup, 3 servings of gelatin, and drank 4 glasses of tea and 3 glasses of juice. To achieve fluid balance, what should Ms. Benjamin's output be?

   ____

CONCLUSION

Mathematical skills are important in determining fluid intake, output, and balance. The skills of addition and comparison are vital in assuring that the health care professional is able to keep a close watch on fluid balance.

REVIEW AND REFLECT

1. Other than intake, what in health care may be estimated?

2. Why is it important to ascertain that intake and output are essentially equal?

3. Why is it important to accurately record intake and output?

4. What math skills are helpful in measuring and comparing intake and output?

5. List some of the dangers of dehydration and overhydration?

UNIT 4

Additional Learning Resources

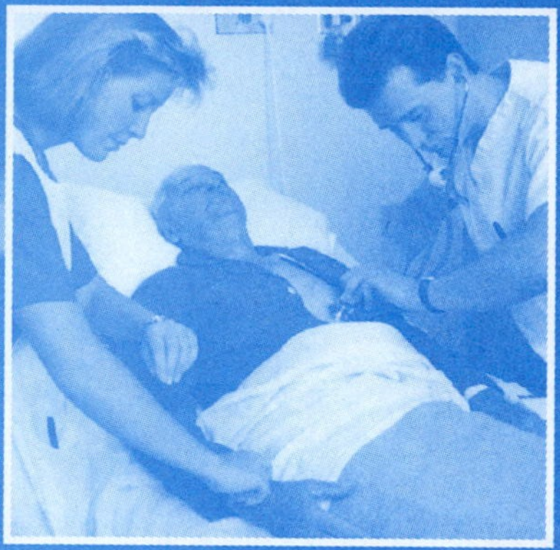

This unit provides a set of resources that will be helpful not only for this class, but also in real life. Knowledge of abbreviations will help save time and assure consistency with other health care professionals, while the equivalency and conversion charts will serve as helpful references both in school and in clinical practice.

The glossary includes all the key terms listed as bold in the text and will serve as a reference for many years. Helpful charts and tables are also provided as a handy reference.

APPENDIX A

Resources

MULTIPLICATION TABLE

X	1	2	3	4	5	6	7	8	9	10	11	12
1	1	2	3	4	5	6	7	8	9	10	11	12
2	2	4	6	8	10	12	14	16	18	20	22	24
3	3	6	9	12	15	18	21	24	27	30	33	36
4	4	8	12	16	20	24	28	32	36	40	44	48
5	5	10	15	20	25	30	35	40	45	50	55	60
6	6	12	18	24	30	36	42	48	54	60	66	72
7	7	14	21	28	35	42	49	56	63	70	77	84
8	8	16	24	32	40	48	56	64	72	80	88	96
9	9	18	27	36	45	54	63	72	81	90	99	108
10	10	20	30	40	50	60	70	80	90	100	110	120
11	11	22	33	44	55	66	77	88	99	110	121	132
12	12	24	36	48	60	72	84	96	108	120	132	144

HEIGHT AND WEIGHT CHARTS

2 to 20 years: Girls
Stature-for-age and Weight-for-age percentiles

NAME ______________

RECORD # __________

Mother's Stature ________ Father's Stature ________

Date	Age	Weight	Stature	BMI*

***To Calculate BMI**: Weight (kg) ÷ Stature (cm) ÷ Stature (cm) x 10,000
or Weight (lb) ÷ Stature (in) ÷ Stature (in) x 703

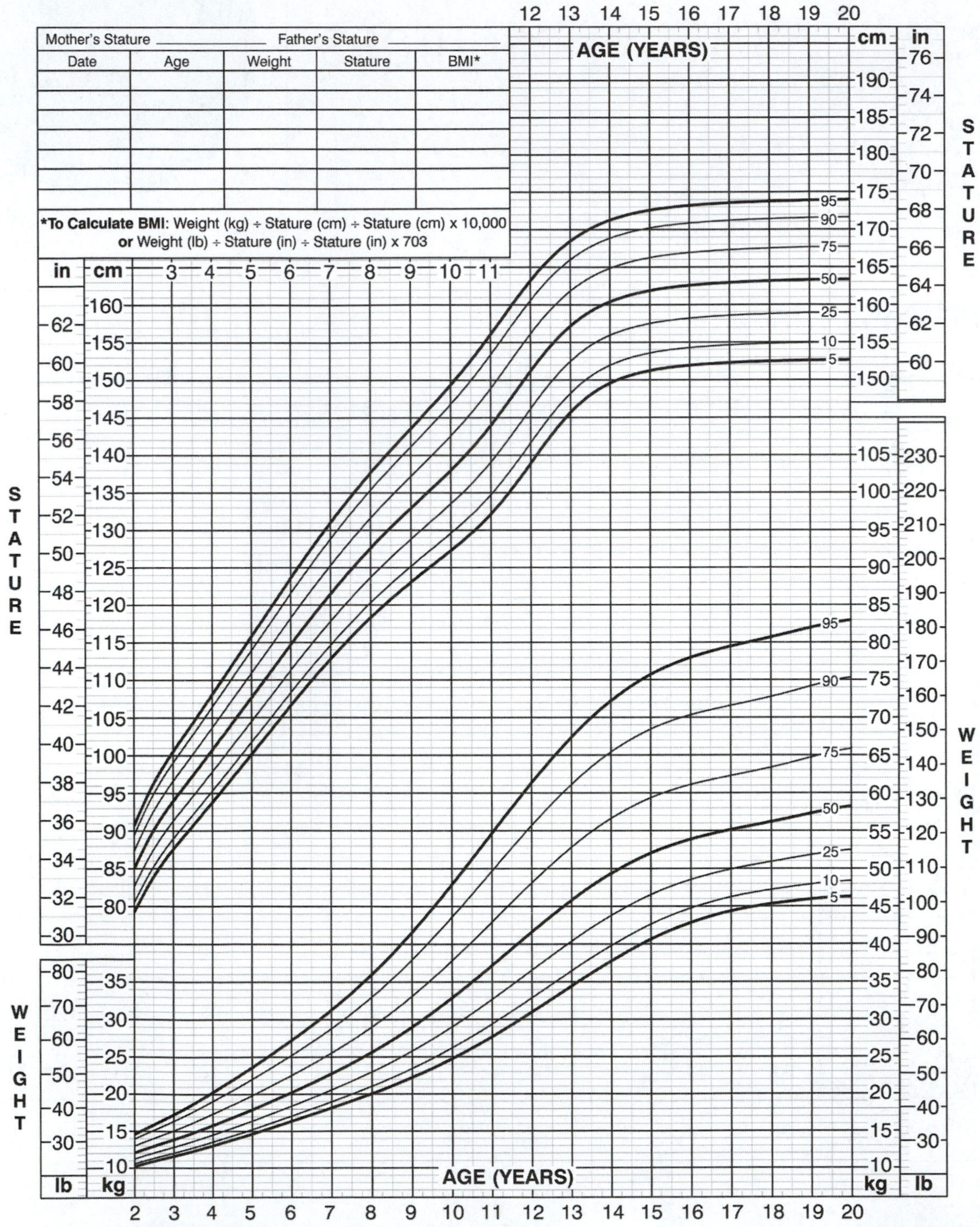

Revised and corrected November 28, 2000.
SOURCE: Developed by the National Center for Health Statistics in collaboration with the National Center for Chronic Disease Prevention and Health Promotion (2000).
http://www.cdc.gov/growthcharts

CDC

HEIGHT AND WEIGHT CHARTS *(continued)*

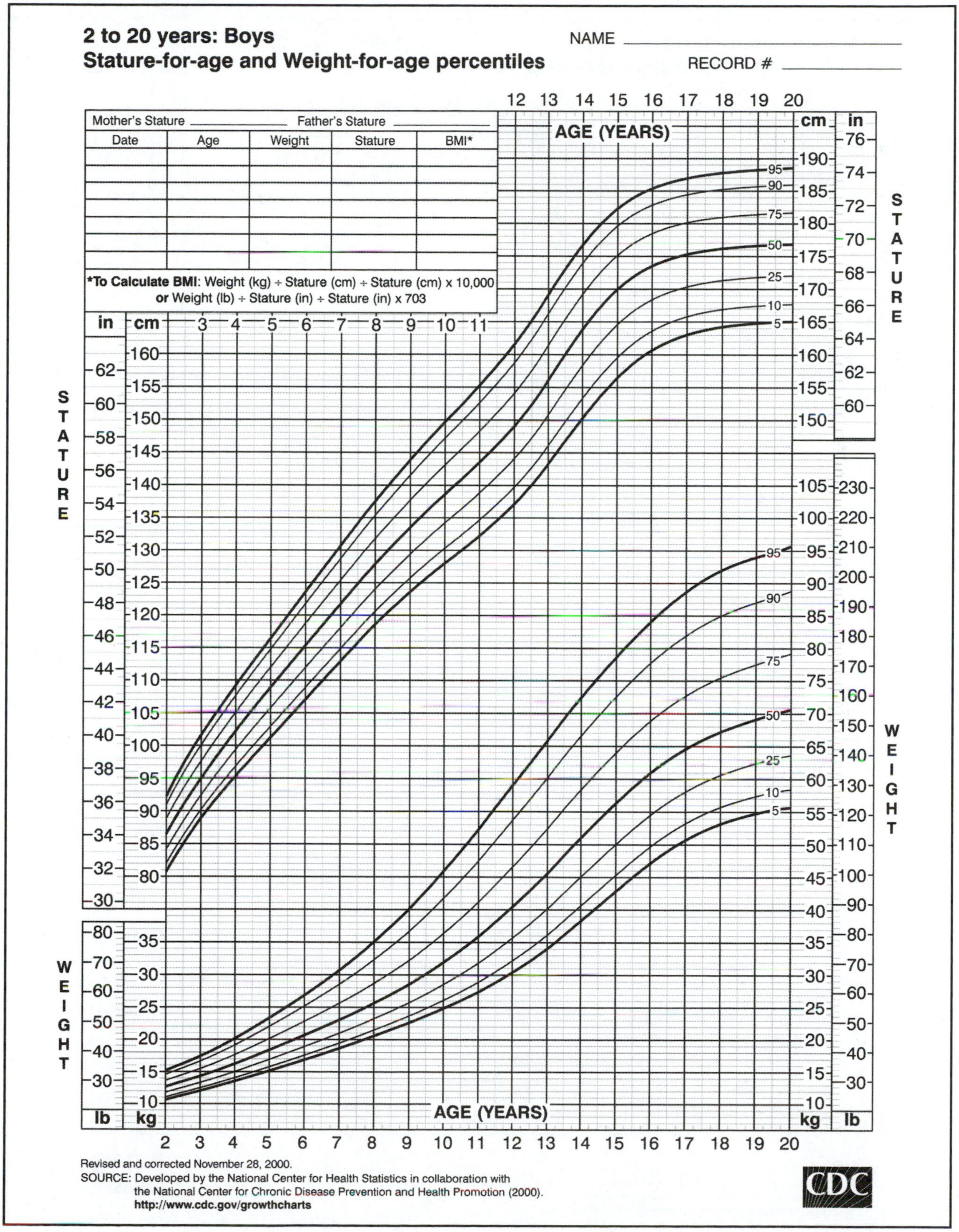

PEDIATRIC GROWTH CHARTS

Birth to 36 months: Girls
Length-for-age and Weight-for-age percentiles

NAME ______________________

RECORD # ____________

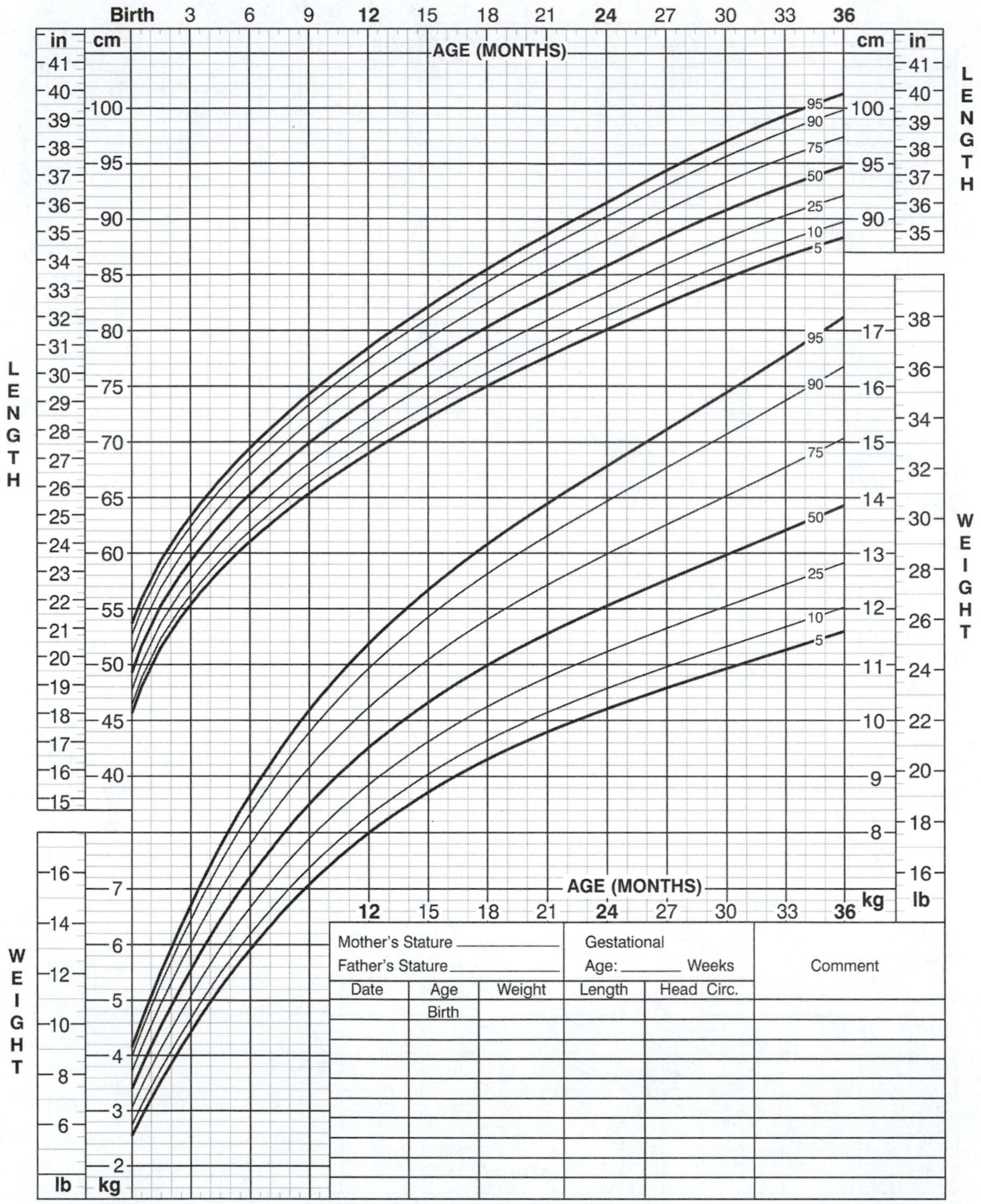

Mother's Stature ________ Father's Stature ________			Gestational Age: ______ Weeks		Comment
Date	Age	Weight	Length	Head Circ.	
	Birth				

Revised April 20, 2001.
SOURCE: Developed by the National Center for Health Statistics in collaboration with the National Center for Chronic Disease Prevention and Health Promotion (2000).
http://www.cdc.gov/growthcharts

PEDIATRIC GROWTH CHARTS *(continued)*

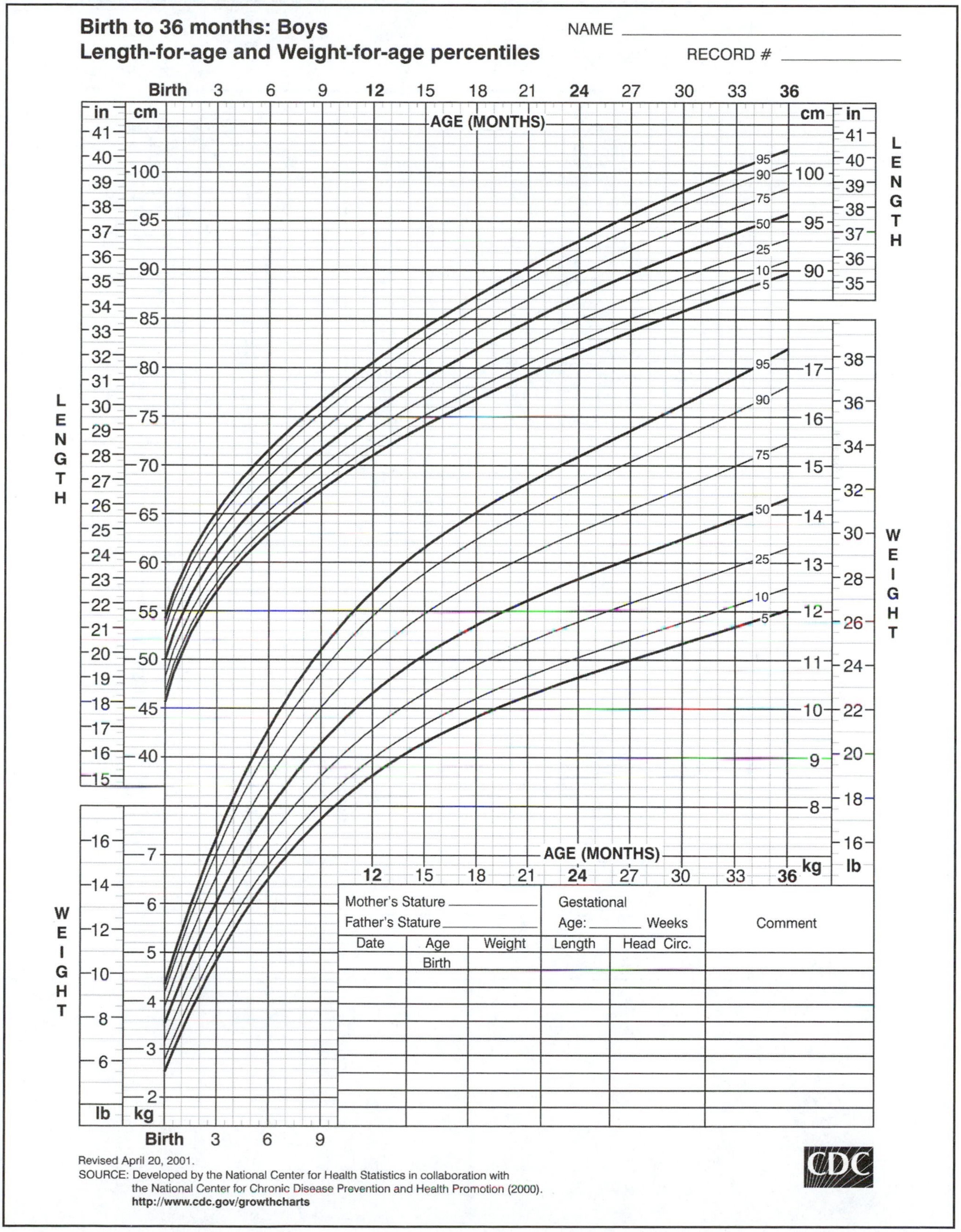

BODY SURFACE AREA NOMOGRAM

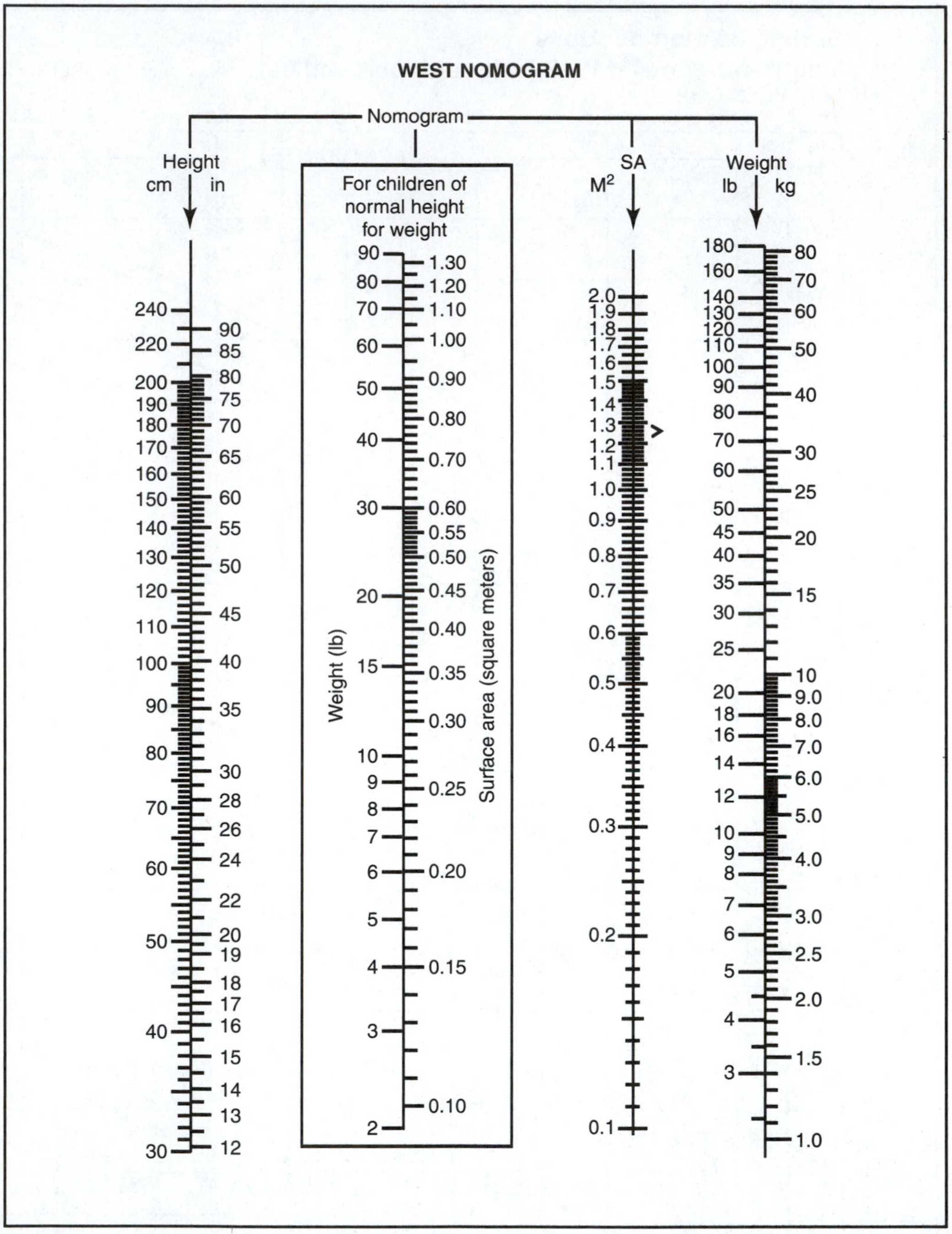

APPENDIX B

Abbreviations

$\bar{a}$	of each
$\overline{aa}$	of each
a.c.	before a meal
alt. dieb.	every other day
alt. hor.	every other hour
alt. noc.	every other night
AM	morning
ap	before dinner
bib.	drink
b.i.d.	twice a day
b.i.n.	twice a night
C	Celsius
$\bar{c}$	with
cap.	capsule
cc	cubic centimeter
cm	centimeter
/d	per day
dr	dram
elix.	elixir
F	Fahrenheit
fldr	fluidram
floz	fluidounce
g	gram
gm	gram
gr	grain
gt	drop
gtt	drop
h	hour
h.d.	at bedtime
hr	hour
h.s.	hour of sleep (bedtime)
IM	intramuscular
inj	injection
I.U.	international unit
kg	kilogram
L	liter
lb	pound
mcg	microgram (μ)
m	meter
m.	minim (♏)
mEq	milliequivalent

mg	milligram
mL	milliliter
mm	millimeter
n.p.o.	nothing by mouth
non. rep.	not to be repeated
o.d.	every day
o.h.	every hour
o.m.	every morning
o.n.	every night
os	mouth
oz	ounce
$\bar{p}$	after
p.c.	after meals
po	by mouth
PM	afternoon or evening
p.r.n.	as needed
pt	pint
q	every
q.d.	every day
q.h.	every hour
q.2h	every 2 hours
q.3h	every 3 hours
q.4h	every 4 hours
q.i.d.	four times a day
q.l.	as much as desired
q.n.	every night
q.o.d.	every other day
q.o.h.	every other hour
q.s.	as much as is required
qt	quart
rep.	let it be repeated
Rx	take thou
$\bar{s}$	without
SC	subcutaneously
Sig.	write on label
SL	sublingual
ss	one half
stat.	immediately
T	temperature
t.i.d.	three times a day
t.i.n.	three times a night
top.	topically
USP	United States Pharmacopeia
ut.dict.	as directed

APPENDIX C

Equivalents

These equivalents are for your reference and provide an approximate, though generally accepted, measure. Frequently-used equivalents should be committed to memory.

LINEAR MEASURE

1 inch = 25.40 millimeters = 2.54 centimeters

1 foot = 12 inches

1 yard = 3 feet

1 meter = 39.37 inches = 3.28 feet = 1.09 yards

1 decameter = 32.81 feet

1 hectometer = 328.08 feet

1 kilometer = 3,280.08 feet = 0.62 mile

1 millimeter = 0.04 inch

1 centimeter = 0.39 inch

1 decimeter = 3.94 inches

WEIGHT

1 pound = 16 ounces

1 kilogram = 2.2 pounds

1 milligram = 0.02 grain

1 centigram = 0.15 grain

1 decigram = 1.54 grains

1 gram = 0.04 ounce

1 decagram = 0.35 ounce

1 hectogram = 3.53 ounces

LIQUID MEASURE

1 tablespoon = 3 teaspoons = 180 drops = 1/2 ounce
1 teaspoon = 60 drops = 1 fluidram
1 fluidounce = 6 teaspoons = 2 tablespoons = 8 fluidrams = 30 milliliters
1 quart = 2 pints = 32 ounces = 1000 milliliters = 4 glasses or cups
1 gallon = 4 quarts = 16 glasses or cups
1 cup = 1 glass = 8 ounces
1 pint = 500 milliliters = 2 glasses or cups = 16 fluidounces
1 medicine cup = 30 milliliters
1 grain = 60 milligrams
1 fluidram = 60 minims = 4 milliliters
1 minim = 1 drop
1 teacup = 6 ounces
1 milliliter = 15 minims

TIME

1 minute = 60 seconds
1 day = 24 hours
1 week = 7 days
1 year = 12 months

DRY MEASURE

1 grain = 60 milligrams
1 gram = 15 grains
1 tablespoon = 15 grams = 4 drams = 3 teaspoons
1 ounce = 30 grams

APPENDIX

Glossary

D

addend—(Chapter 4) In addition, the numbers that are added.

apothecary system—(Chapter 3) Measurement system that is used on a limited basis.

average—(Chapter 4) A mathematical mean found by adding a list of numbers and dividing by the number in the set.

body surface area (BSA)—(Chapter 11) A mathematical estimate, expressed in square meters (m^2), used to calculate medication dosages, usually in children.

borrow—(Chapter 4) When subtracting, what you do when the digit you are subtracting is greater than the digit you are subtracting from. You must move, or borrow, a digit from the place to the immediate left, allowing you to subtract.

canceling—(Chapter 6) Finding the product of two fractions by reducing fractions.

Celsius—(Chapter 11) The international thermometric scale in which 0° is freezing and 100° is boiling.

common denominator—(Chapter 6) Denominators that are the same number.

common factor—(Chapter 6) A factor that belongs to two or more numbers.

concentration of a solution—(Chapter 10) The amount of solute that has been dissolved in a specific amount of fluid.

conversion—(Chapter 9) The act of changing from one system or measurement to another.

decimal—(Chapter 5) A fraction of a whole number whose denominators are multiples of 10.

dehydration—(Chapter 12) A fluid imbalance in which fluid is deficient.

denominator—(Chapter 6) The number of parts by which an item is divided. It is shown as the bottom number in a fraction.

difference—(Chapter 4) In subtraction, the answer.

dividend—(Chapter 4) In division, the number being divided.

divisor—(Chapter 4) In division, the number divided into the dividend.

drip rate—(Chapter 10) The rate in which the fluid drips from the intravenous bag into the intravenous line.

English system—(Chapter 3) Synonym for household system of measurement.

expiration date—(Chapter 10) The last date in which a medication should be used.

extremes—(Chapter 7) The end, or outside components, of a proportion.

factor—(Chapter 4) In multiplication, the numbers being multiplied.

Fahrenheit—(Chapter 11) The thermometric scale in which 32° is freezing and 212° is boiling.

fraction—(Chapter 6) A part of a whole.

generic name—(Chapter 10) Nonproprietary name of a medication.

greatest common factor (GCF)—(Chapter 6) The largest factor that two or more numbers have in common.

hard skills—(Chapter 1) Set of job requirements that require technical expertise. For example, starting an IV or assessing a blood pressure.

Hindu-Arabic system—(Chapter 2) A numerical system developed approximately 600 A.D. in India by the Hindus and brought to the Western world by the Arabs. It is sometimes referred to as the Arabic system.

household system—(Chapter 3) System of measurement that utilizes measuring devices that are readily available in most homes. Prescribed medications are frequently converted to household measures.

improper fraction—(Chapter 6) A fraction in which the numerator is greater than the denominator.

intake—(Chapter 12) That which is taken into the body.

KVO line—(Chapter 10) Keep vein open. Designation for intravenous drip rate that runs as a rate sufficient to keep a line open for medication administration.

least common denominator (LCD)—(Chapter 6) The lowest number into which all the denominators in a set can be divided.

least common multiple (LCM)—(Chapter 6) The smallest multiple that is shared by two or more numbers.

lot number—(Chapter 10) Internal reference number used by a manufacturer so that medications may be traced to the day and the batch in which they were manufactured.

macrodrip—(Chapter 10) Drip set commonly used for fluid replacement and/or to keep a route available for intravenous medications; commonly available in 10, 12, or 15 drops per mL. Also referred to as a standard drip set.

mean—(Chapter 4) A mathematical average found by adding all the numbers in a set and dividing the sum by the quantity of the set.

means—(Chapter 7) The middle components of a proportion.

medication label—(Chapter 10) A label that contains important information to help the health care professional deliver the right medication to the patient. Components of the medication label include trade name, generic name, manufacturer, NDC number, dosage strength, drug form, usual adult dose, total amount enclosed, prescription warning, expiration date, and lot number.

metric system—(Chapter 3) A decimal system of weights and measures based on the meter, liter, and gram.

microdrip—(Chapter 10) Intravenous drip set used when volume must be limited. A microdrip set delivers one mL for every 60 drops of fluid that drips through the set.

minuend—(Chapter 4) In subtraction, the number from which you subtract.

mixed number—(Chapter 6) A combination consisting of a whole number and a fraction.

multiple—(Chapter 6) The product of a whole number multiplied by a whole number.

multiplicand—(Chapter 4) In multiplication, the number being multiplied.

multiplier—(Chapter 4) In multiplication, the number by which the multiplicand is being multiplied.

nomogram—(Chapter 11) A graphic image in which a straight line connects known values to find an unknown value; sometimes used to measure body surface area and children's height and weight.

numerator—(Chapter 6) The number of parts represented in the fraction. It is shown as the top number in the fraction.

numerical system—(Chapter 2) An organized system for counting.

output—(Chapter 12) Liquid that is excreted from the body.

overhydration—(Chapter 12) A fluid imbalance in which there is an excess of fluids.

percent (%)—(Chapter 8) A part of one hundred.

percent strength—(Chapter 10) Refers to the percentage of a solvent in a given solute.

piggyback—(Chapter 10) A medication infusion that is attached to an already existing (primary) IV line.

place value—(Chapter 4) The value of a digit specified by its location in relation to the decimal.

prescription—(Chapter 10) A medication order that a physician writes or telephones to a pharmacy.

product—(Chapter 4) In multiplication, the result.

proper fraction—(Chapter 6) A fraction in which the denominator is greater than the numerator.

proportion—(Chapter 7) An equation that states that two ratios are equal.

quotient—(Chapter 4) In division, the dividend divided by the divisor is the quotient.

ratio—(Chapter 7) A comparison of numbers by division.

remainder—(Chapter 4) In division, if there is part of the dividend that is not divided, it is called the remainder.

Roman numerals—(Chapter 2) An additive system created by ancient Romans. This system is thought to have evolved from tick marks on the ground and is still used on a limited basis today. Numbers are read by adding and/or subtracting a series of symbols.

soft skills—(Chapter 1) Set of foundational job requirements that may not require specific technical skills, but instead focus on general job preparation. Examples include mathematics, communication skills, and reading for information.

subtrahend—(Chapter 4) In subtraction, the number to be subtracted.

sum—(Chapter 4) The total of a series of added numbers.

syringe—(Chapter 10) Graduated cylindrical container that is used to administer precise amounts of medication.

terms—(Chapter 7) The numbers that are compared in a ratio.

TKO line—(Chapter 10) To keep open. Designation for intravenous drip rate that runs as a rate sufficient to keep a line open for medication administration.

trade name—(Chapter 10) The proprietary name of a medication, usually protected by a trademark.

uncommon denominator—(Chapter 6) Denominators that are not the same.

uncommon factor— (Chapter 6) Factors that are not common to two or more numbers.

whole number—(Chapter 4) Any of the set of nonnegative integers.

APPENDIX E

Final Summative Evaluation

Answer each of the following problems.

You are asked to weigh and measure a new patient in your unit. When you weight Mrs. Ahsirt, you note the following reading.

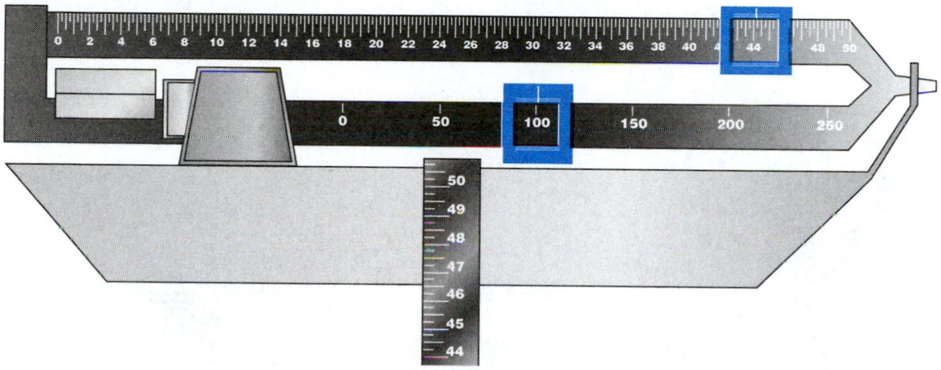

You note Mrs. Ahsirt's height on the rule below.

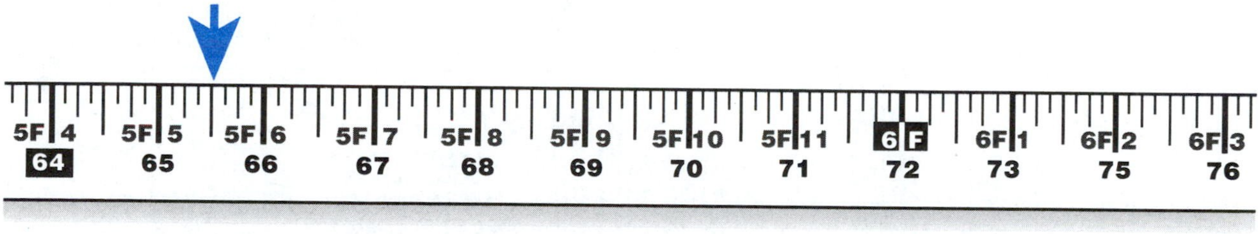

1. What is Mrs. Ahsirt's weight in pounds?

____

2. What is Mrs. Ahsirt's height in English measurement?

____

Mrs. Ahsirt's orders include the following:

MEDICATION	DOSAGE	ROUTE	FREQ
Cephalexin cap.	500 mg	PO	q6h

3. Check the box of the correct medications.

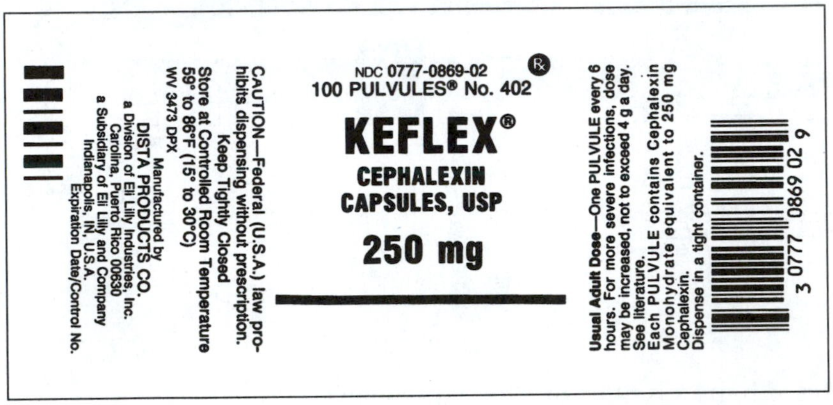

☐ A

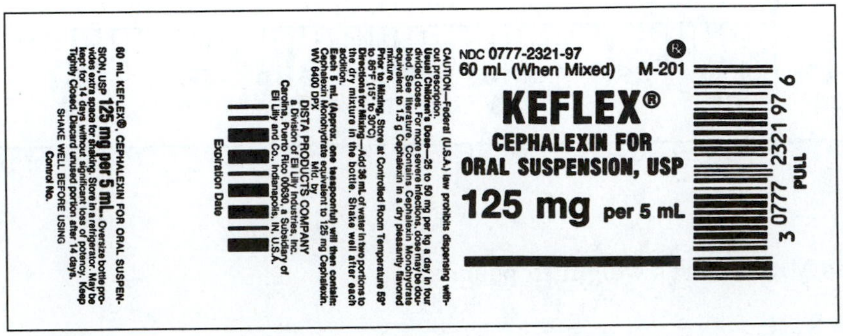

☐ B

☐ Both labels are correct.

☐ Neither label is correct.

4. How many capsules will you administer?

____

5. How frequently will this medicine be administered?

____

6. What is the trade name of this medication?

____

7. Who is the manufacturer of this medication?

____

Another patient, Mr. Genheim, has the following order written on his chart.

MEDICATION	DOSAGE	ROUTE	FREQ
Furosemide	*80 mg*	*iv*	*non. rep.*

You locate the following medication in your medicine room.

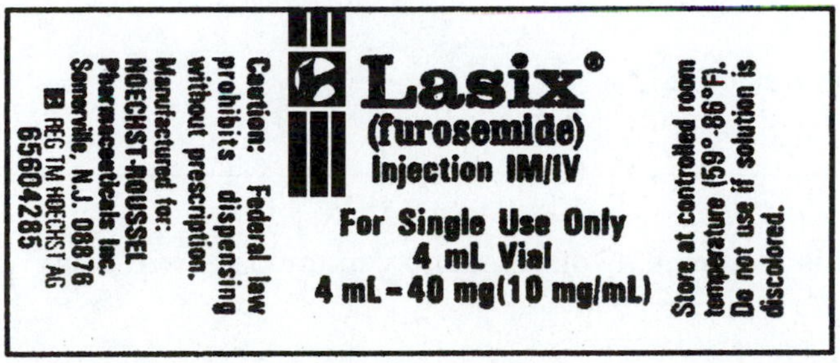

8. What is the trade name for this medicine?

____

9. How many mL do you administer?

____

10. How often will this dose be administered?

____

A pharmacist receives the following prescription for Mrs. Brown.

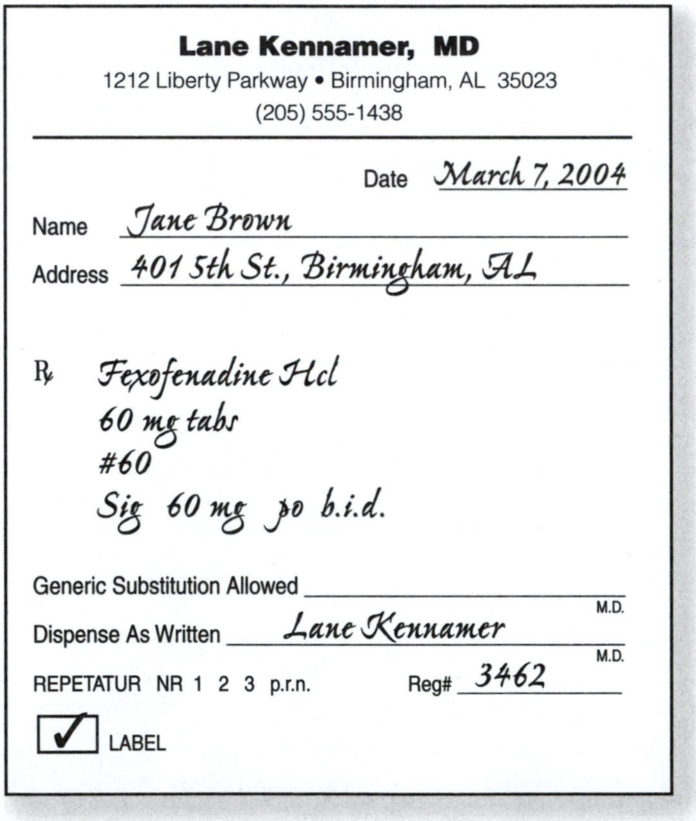

Lane Kennamer, MD
1212 Liberty Parkway • Birmingham, AL 35023
(205) 555-1438

Date *March 7, 2004*

Name *Jane Brown*

Address *401 5th St., Birmingham, AL*

℞ *Fexofenadine Hcl*
60 mg tabs
#60
Sig 60 mg po b.i.d.

Generic Substitution Allowed ______________ M.D.

Dispense As Written *Lane Kennamer* M.D.

REPETATUR NR 1 2 3 p.r.n. Reg# *3462*

☑ LABEL

11. How many tablets are prescribed?

____

12. If the patient takes this medicine as directed, how many days will this prescription last?

____

13. This medicine should be stored at a temperature of between 20°C to 25°C. In Fahrenheit, what temperature range should this medicine be kept?

____

Your patient has consumed the following:

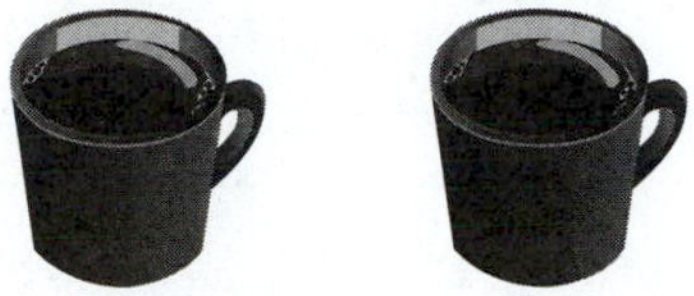

2 cups of coffee

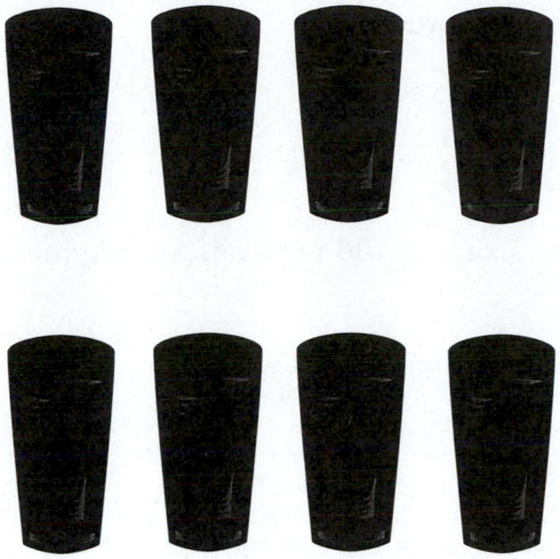

8 glasses of water

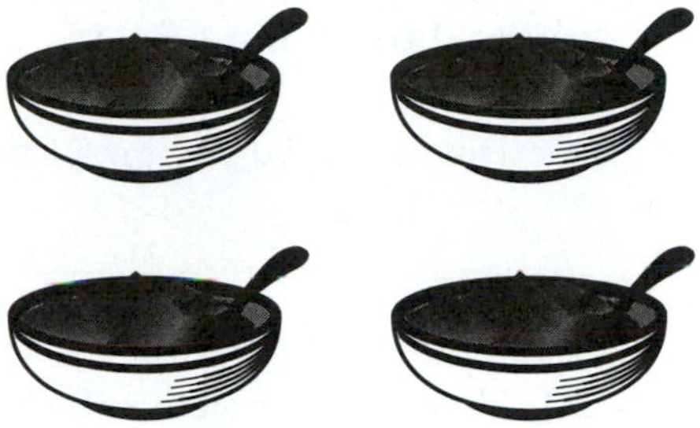

4 bowls of gelatin

14. Estimate this patient's intake.

____

15. What would you expect this patient's output to be?

____

You are asked to start an intravenous line on Mr. Linden. The physician asks you to administer 600 mL of lactated ringers over 4 hours.

16. Circle the most appropriate drip set.

a. Microdrip (60 drop set)

b. Macrodrip (10 drop set)

17. Based on the drip set that you chose in question 17, at what rate would you run the IV?

____

18. Your unit stocks 500 mL bags of lactated ringers. At the ordered rate, how quickly will the 500 mL bag empty?

____

19. What percentage of the second 500 mL bag will be administered to the patient to comply with the physician's orders?

____

20. You are asked to administer Lorazepam, 3mg to your patient. Lorazepam is supplied in 0.5 mg, 1 mg, and 2 mg tablets. What combination of these tablets would you administer to attain the ordered dose?

____

Your patient's prescription calls for Amoxapine 100 mg t.i.d. Amoxapine is supplied in 50 mg tablets.

21. How often do you direct the patient to take his medicine?

____

22. How many tablets will the patient take to meet his 100 mg dose?

____

23. After three days, the patient calls you to inform you that he believes he has missed one or more doses of his medicine. Assuming that he has taken the appropriate number of doses each of the three days since his prescription was filled, how many tablets should the patient have taken so far?

____

24. You are asked to administer 4,000 units of Botulinum Toxin, Type B to your patient. This medication is supplied 5,000 units/mL. How many mL will you administer?

____

25. You need to administer 5 mg/kg of Bretylium tosylate to your patient, who weighs 195 lbs. Bretylium is supplied 50 mg/mL. How many mL will you administer?

____

ANSWERS TO SELECTED QUESTIONS

CHAPTER 1 MATH AS A HEALTH CARE FUNCTION

Self-Assessment Pretest

Answers require a personal response.

CHAPTER 2 NUMERICAL SYSTEMS

Self-Assessment Pretest

1. 4
2. 12
3. 1,154
4. 5
5. 8
6. 36
7. 19
8. 190
9. 1,983
10. 1,965
11. MMIII
12. XIV
13. XCVIII
14. MMMCDLVI
15. CCXXXI
16. DCCXCVIII
17. CDLXV
18. II
19. LXXII
20. CXII

Objective 2.2 Skill Sharpener

1. 26
3. 601
5. 138
7. 2,000
9. 24

Objective 2.3 Skill Sharpener

1. CVL
3. CCCXII
5. MCCCXCIV
7. XXXVIII
9. MMMCCXVII

CHAPTER 3 MEASUREMENT SYSTEMS

Self-Assessment Pretest

1. A
2. C
3. B
4. C
5. A
6. B
7. A
8. B
9. A
10. B

Objective 3.2 Skill Sharpener

Apothecary System of Weight

1. 3 gr
3. 8 oz or 8℥
5. $\frac{1}{200}$ gr
7. 3 oz or 3℥
9. 2 lb 11 oz or 2 lb 11℥

Apothecary System of Volume

1. 4 ♏ or 4 m
3. 3 floz
5. 2 qt
7. 2 m or 2 ♏
9. 5 fldr or 5ʒ

Objective 3.4 Skill Sharpener

Prefixes

1. $\frac{1}{10}$ or 0.1
3. 1000
5. $\frac{1}{1000}$ or 0.001
7. $\frac{1}{100}$ or 0.01

Metric Units of Measure

	Measure of	Multiple or fraction
1.	length	fraction
3.	length	multiple
5.	weight	fraction
7.	volume	fraction
9.	weight	multiple

CHAPTER 4 WHOLE NUMBER REVIEW

Self-Assessment Pretest

1. 23
2. 543
3. 78
4. 93
5. 1
6. 34
7. 998
8. 3,292
9. 56,732
10. 750

11. 124
12. 376
13. 89,977
14. 4,965
15. 324
16. 10,922
17. 300
18. 12
19. 13,545
20. 10
21. 123
22. 9,878
23. 13,243
24. 45,878
25. 990
26. 765
27. 78,900
28. 200
29. 43,342
30. 65,400
31. 12,390
32. 78,980
33. 32,534
34. 1,200
35. 9,878
36. 45,000
37. 123,000
38. 454,302
39. 500,954
40. 231,493
41. 14,390
42. 54,322
43. 299,987
44. 298,773
45. 12,098
46. 34,094
47. 150,900
48. 54,000
49. 893,204
50. 434,000
51. 756,321
52. 1,235,434
53. 34,343,665
54. 1,200,900
55. 2,987,655
56. 45,443,345
57. 656,999
58. 2,124,000
59. 456,222
60. 9,000,000
61. <
62. <
63. =
64. <
65. >
66. >
67. <
68. =
69. =
70. >
71. 100, 1234, 34323, 54323
72. 343, 657, 659, 787
73. 454, 654, 656, 7676
74. 112, 121, 211, 222
75. 342, 343, 454, 544
76. 343, 345, 346, 365
77. 394, 493, 873, 878
78. 300, 382, 394, 398
79. 482, 483, 849, 940
80. 345, 433, 493, 984
81. 460
82. 7,600
83. 880
84. 910
85. 1,290
86. 330
87. 760
88. 900
89. 400
90. 430
91. 3,500
92. 54,500
93. 34,700
94. 1,200
95. 78,600
96. 23,000
97. 4,300
98. 55,500
99. 98,900
100. 430,000
101. 34,000
102. 94,000
103. 43,000
104. 76,000
105. 99,000
106. 54,000
107. 45,000
108. 79,000
109. 75,000
110. 494,000
111. 14
112. 68
113. 999
114. 1,280
115. 113,342
116. 4,318,306
117. 12,745
118. 444,284
119. 450,452
120. 46,610,526
121. 380
122. 245
123. 11,587
124. 16,576
125. 27,895
126. 242,759
127. 65
128. 423
129. 1,222
130. 6,001
131. 46
132. 7,854
133. 377,136
134. 529,760
135. 934,017
136. 1,027,043
137. 330,261,672
138. 606,339
139. 62,000
140. 25,056
141. 5
142. 5
143. 15 with remainder of 39
144. 21 with remainder of 15
145. 28 with remainder of 2
146. 260 with remainder of 273
147. 2,620
148. 208 with remainder of 120
149. 4
150. 58
151. 8.6
152. 16.2
153. 437.4
154. 69.67
155. 720
156. 8138.6
157. 70.67
158. 34
159. 508.4
160. 96.375

Objective 4.2 Skill Sharpener

1. 34,506
3. 123
5. 5,463
7. 912
9. 987
11. 34,506
13. 123
15. 5,463
17. 912
19. 987
21. 34,506
23. 123
25. 5,463
27. 912
29. 987
31. 34,506
33. 123,243
35. 5,443
37. 9,182
39. 98,701
41. 34,506
43. 123,900
45. 55,443
47. 95,212
49. 987,000
51. hundreds
53. ones
55. tens
57. thousands
59. ten thousands

Objective 4.3 Skill Sharpener

1. <
3. <
5. <
7. =
9. <

Objective 4.4 Skill Sharpener

1. 1, 3, 23, 32, 54
3. 4, 34, 35, 41, 43
5. 3, 6, 34, 54, 76
7. 1, 3, 23, 54, 456
9. 3, 4, 34, 43, 343

Objective 4.5 Skill Sharpener

1. 10
3. 850
5. 100
7. 910
9. 80
11. 1,300
13. 500
15. 800
17. 500
19. 100
21. 46,000
23. 3,000
25. 191,000
27. 1,000
29. 398,000
31. 343,838,837,120
33. 343,838,837,000
35. 343,838,800,000
37. 343,840,000,000
39. 344,000,000,000

Objective 4.6 Skill Sharpener

1. 147
3. 13,239
5. 13
7. 533
9. 555
11. 2,628
13. 1,571
15. 6,634
17. 2,356
19. 4,322

Objective 4.7 Skill Sharpener

1. 9
3. 953
5. 757,555
7. 958
9. 7,285,910

Objective 4.8 Skill Sharpener

1. 408
3. 102,810
5. 23,190,609,204
7. 176,400
9. 39,583,516

Objective 4.9 Skill Sharpener

1. 6
3. 835 with remainder of 113
5. 183 with remainder of 59
7. 130
9. 247 with remainder of 78

Objective 4.10 Skill Sharpener

1. 93
2. 149.34
3. 239.2
4. 1086.4
5. 906.8
6. 89
7. 13,032.34
8. 2,800.34
9. 4815.67

CHAPTER 5 DECIMALS

Self-Assessment Pretest

1. 45.34
2. 690.00
3. 212.932
4. 32.893
5. 785.112
6. 3215.190
7. 9950.250
8. 451.364
9. 34590.773
10. 23321.500
11. 54.980
12. 6790.3532
13. 356.121
14. 100.56
15. 4341.5550
16. 67650.341
17. 900.9000
18. 15250.375
19. 8.375
20. 100.875
21. 34.1230
22. 500.3209
23. 65.9010
24. 750.8793
25. 3500.5300
26. 353.1250
27. 795.975
28. 900.01991
29. 63475.9801

30. 7601.9000
31. 540.3421
32. 442.3928
33. 7988.8897
34. 452.5203
35. 32321.9002
36. 431.23179
37. 299.2020
38. 29.20232
39. 365.245
40. 943.7075
41. <
42. =
43. =
44. <
45. >
46. >
47. >
48. =
49. <
50. =
51. 34.3
52. 12.4
53. 453.9
54. 45.4
55. 475.8
56. 939.3
57. 948.4
58. 397.3
59. 94847.9
60. 948.5
61. 8347.47
62. 34.32
63. 455.45
64. 499.96
65. 595.59
66. 4.45
67. 45.44
68. 995.55
69. 454.44
70. 9045.44
71. 3433.334
72. 44.404
73. 434.444
74. 8.645
75. 0.333
76. 102.233
77. 3.343
78. 6.454
79. 4.540
80. 9.405
81. 377.55
82. 486.33
83. 1227.765
84. 54.776
85. 354346.6984
86. 1441.73
87. 9902.833
88. 99665.39509
89. 808.64
90. 972.4
91. 33.989
92. 3.107
93. 431.48157
94. 0.94
95. 56.013
96. 9427.92
97. 9.999
98. 0.31
99. 5908.972
100. 1.99
101. 70229.28
102. 110.166
103. 178425584.8
104. 422671555.8
105. 369771.9048
106. 73.38
107. 7093150.641
108. 893703.66
109. 6655.11
110. 3191.76
111. 3.726708075
112. 1.524805147
113. 1.361797753
114. 8.507175573
115. 12.41090343
116. 2.50352786
117. 19.07960326
118. 1.133545873
119. 24.28338335
120. 4.721718806
121. 318.1814
122. 152.7266
123. 91.21825
124. 514.9855
125. 900.6344
126. 126.2412
127. 9.7754
128. 4.4998
129. 82.832
130. 4.73322

Objective 5.2 Skill Sharpener

1. 12300
3. 21938
5. 2222222
7. 3467
9. 12789
11. 56.9987
13. 9292.77382
15. 993.909
17. 758.423
19. 9832.9853
21. 8437.0303
23. 487.0932
25. 4576.888
27. 8594.90329
29. 982.030908
31. 637367.8969
33. 895.2090
35. 0009.00009
37. 8578.9834
39. 3298398.9696

Objective 5.3 Skill Sharpener

1. 175.98
3. 99,349.67
5. 17.7631
7. $3,943.32
9. $3,060.53

Objective 5.4 Skill Sharpener

1. >
3. >
5. <
7. =
9. =

Objective 5.5 Skill Sharpener

1. 843.8
3. 728.9
5. 13.4
7. 574837.4
9. 84398.8
11. 8437.48
13. 22.22

15. 4903.70
17. 9303.31
19. 302.94
21. 78.939
23. 93939.066
25. 8439.524
27. 098.433
29. 998432497.585

Objective 5.6 Skill Sharpener

1. 12.9
3. 166.78
5. 579.62
7. 31.9
9. 9489.078

Objective 5.7 Skill Sharpener

1. 2.4
3. 4556.9
5. 6583.302
7. 1111.1
9. 9.92

Objective 5.8 Skill Sharpener

1. 76094.6736
3. 881898.792
5. 4637144.314
7. 41579.2356
9. 6768770.112

Objective 5.9 Skill Sharpener

1. 1420.464
3. 30.7
5. 3.014876
7. 10
9. 97.125

Objective 5.10 Skill Sharpener

1. 6.45
3. $4.\overline{33}$
5. 19.14
7. 54.675
9. 7.58

CHAPTER 6 FRACTIONS

Self-Assessment Pretest

1. $\frac{1}{2}$
2. $\frac{23}{48}$
3. $\frac{2}{10}$
4. $\frac{6}{12}$
5. $\frac{125}{1000}$
6. $\frac{15}{90}$
7. $\frac{2}{900}$
8. $\frac{45}{500}$
9. $\frac{6}{9}$
10. $\frac{180}{360}$
11. $\frac{12}{14}$
12. $\frac{5}{61}$
13. $\frac{15}{16}$
14. $\frac{7}{8}$
15. $\frac{3}{4}$
16. $\frac{325}{650}$
17. $\frac{9}{12}$
18. $\frac{500}{15000}$
19. $\frac{4}{16}$
20. $\frac{17}{18}$
21. $\frac{1}{6}$ $\frac{1}{5}$ $\frac{1}{4}$ $\frac{1}{3}$ $\frac{1}{2}$
22. $\frac{3}{8}$ $\frac{7}{16}$ $\frac{1}{2}$ $\frac{9}{16}$ $\frac{3}{4}$
23. $\frac{11}{16}$ $\frac{12}{16}$ $\frac{12}{15}$ $\frac{7}{8}$ $\frac{9}{10}$
24. $\frac{6}{15}$ $\frac{4}{9}$ $\frac{3}{4}$ $\frac{4}{5}$ $\frac{10}{12}$
25. $\frac{1}{2}$ $\frac{2}{3}$ $\frac{3}{4}$ $\frac{4}{5}$ $\frac{5}{6}$
26. $\frac{7}{64}$ $\frac{3}{16}$ $\frac{9}{32}$ $\frac{5}{8}$ $\frac{6}{8}$
27. $\frac{9}{14}$ $\frac{2}{3}$ $\frac{13}{16}$ $\frac{7}{8}$ $\frac{15}{16}$
28. $\frac{2}{45}$ $\frac{5}{75}$ $\frac{4}{7}$ $\frac{9}{15}$ $\frac{4}{5}$
29. $\frac{9}{16}$ $\frac{2}{3}$ $\frac{12}{15}$ $\frac{13}{16}$ $\frac{7}{8}$
30. $\frac{8}{100}$ $\frac{3}{8}$ $\frac{8}{12}$ $\frac{16}{24}$ $\frac{4}{5}$
31. 1
32. 1
33. $1\frac{1}{16}$
34. $\frac{5}{12}$
35. $\frac{9}{32}$
36. $\frac{4}{5}$
37. $\frac{11}{20}$
38. $\frac{24}{25}$
39. $\frac{3}{4}$
40. $\frac{1}{12}$
41. $\frac{1}{50}$
42. $\frac{1}{4}$
43. $\frac{3}{10}$
44. $\frac{1}{2}$
45. $\frac{2}{5}$
46. $\frac{1}{2}$
47. $\frac{1}{10}$
48. $\frac{5}{6}$
49. $\frac{143}{600}$
50. $\frac{2}{5}$
51. 4
52. $4\frac{1}{8}$
53. 28
54. 19
55. $5\frac{1}{2}$
56. $6\frac{1}{2}$
57. $53\frac{3}{4}$
58. $10\frac{2}{9}$
59. $5\frac{7}{9}$
60. $36\frac{77}{90}$
61. $10\frac{1}{2}$
62. $53\frac{1}{2}$
63. $\frac{3}{16}$
64. $36\frac{5}{8}$
65. $10\frac{4}{5}$
66. $3\frac{3}{4}$
67. $29\frac{2}{3}$
68. $3\frac{43}{50}$
69. $4\frac{4}{7}$
70. $4\frac{5}{8}$
71. 1, 2, 3, 4, 6, 12
72. 1, 2, 4, 8, 16
73. 1, 2, 3, 6
74. 1, 2, 5, 10
75. 1, 2, 4, 8
76. 1, 2, 7, 14
77. 1, 2, 4, 8, 16, 32
78. 1, 7
79. 1, 2, 4
80. 1, 2, 3, 6, 9, 18
81. 6
82. 6
83. 3
84. 8
85. 4
86. 2
87. 4
88. 9
89. 4
90. 12
91. $\frac{1}{2}$
92. $\frac{1}{3}$
93. $\frac{1}{16}$
94. $\frac{1}{3}$
95. $\frac{7}{8}$
96. $\frac{5}{8}$
97. $\frac{9}{10}$
98. $\frac{4}{5}$
99. $\frac{1}{3}$

100. $\frac{3}{5}$
101. $\frac{2}{1}$ or 2
102. $\frac{4}{1}$ or 4
103. $1\frac{2}{5}$
104. $\frac{4}{1}$ or 4
105. $\frac{9}{1}$ or 9
106. $1\frac{1}{3}$
107. $1\frac{1}{6}$
108. $\frac{6}{1}$ or 6
109. $\frac{15}{1}$ or 15
110. $1\frac{1}{2}$
111. 12
112. 9
113. 14
114. 20
115. 10
116. 150
117. 49
118. 12
119. 8
120. 32
121. 12
122. 48
123. 24
124. 48
125. 20
126. 72
127. 120
128. 72
129. 24
130. 24
131. $\frac{11}{12}$
132. $1\frac{1}{2}$
133. $1\frac{5}{14}$
134. $1\frac{2}{15}$
135. $\frac{13}{16}$
136. $1\frac{1}{9}$
137. $1\frac{1}{18}$
138. $1\frac{11}{40}$
139. $1\frac{8}{35}$
140. $1\frac{15}{18}$
141. $\frac{13}{24}$
142. $\frac{11}{24}$
143. $\frac{1}{6}$
144. $\frac{7}{12}$
145. $\frac{3}{16}$
146. $\frac{1}{3}$
147. $\frac{5}{18}$
148. $\frac{17}{30}$
149. $\frac{1}{8}$
150. $\frac{3}{4}$
151. $1\frac{3}{4}$
152. $3\frac{2}{3}$
153. $\frac{7}{8}$
154. $3\frac{2}{5}$
155. $1\frac{7}{8}$
156. $1\frac{1}{2}$
157. $3\frac{13}{16}$
158. $1\frac{3}{4}$
159. $1\frac{3}{4}$
160. $1\frac{4}{5}$
161. $\frac{9}{8}$
162. $\frac{33}{9}$
163. $\frac{7}{2}$
164. $\frac{51}{4}$
165. $\frac{21}{8}$
166. $\frac{11}{5}$
167. $\frac{29}{6}$
168. $\frac{28}{16}$
169. $\frac{49}{12}$
170. $\frac{15}{4}$
171. $\frac{1}{2}$
172. $\frac{5}{12}$
173. $\frac{3}{10}$
174. $\frac{5}{12}$
175. $\frac{21}{32}$
176. $\frac{7}{20}$
177. $\frac{2}{9}$
178. $\frac{2}{9}$
179. $\frac{7}{10}$
180. $\frac{3}{4}$
181. 8
182. $1\frac{1}{2}$
183. $2\frac{3}{16}$
184. $1\frac{3}{4}$
185. $\frac{45}{64}$
186. $1\frac{4}{5}$
187. $2\frac{1}{2}$
188. $42\frac{7}{8}$
189. $1\frac{11}{25}$
190. $4\frac{1}{8}$
191. $1\frac{1}{8}$
192. $1\frac{1}{2}$
193. $1\frac{19}{21}$
194. $1\frac{7}{8}$
195. $1\frac{5}{16}$
196. $1\frac{2}{5}$
197. $13\frac{1}{3}$
198. $3\frac{11}{15}$
199. 5
200. 2

Objective 6.3 Skill Sharpener

1. $\frac{1}{2}$
3. $\frac{12}{32}$
5. $\frac{9}{10}$
7. $\frac{3}{4}$
9. $\frac{10}{12}$

Objective 6.4 Skill Sharpener

1. $\frac{3}{4}$
3. $\frac{1}{2}$
5. $\frac{17}{32}$
7. $\frac{3}{8}$
9. $\frac{22}{100}$

Objective 6.5 Skill Sharpener

1. $\frac{2}{5}$ $\frac{5}{8}$ $\frac{2}{3}$
3. $\frac{1}{5}$ $\frac{1}{2}$ $\frac{3}{4}$
5. $\frac{1}{5}$ $\frac{3}{6}$ $\frac{2}{3}$
7. $\frac{1}{8}$ $\frac{2}{6}$ $\frac{2}{3}$
9. $\frac{6}{7}$ $\frac{7}{8}$ $\frac{8}{9}$

Objective 6.6 Skill Sharpener

1. $1\frac{2}{5}$
3. $\frac{7}{8}$
5. $\frac{5}{9}$
7. $1\frac{1}{8}$
9. $\frac{9}{10}$

Objective 6.7 Skill Sharpener

1. $\frac{1}{2}$
3. $\frac{1}{3}$
5. $\frac{27}{50}$
7. $\frac{9}{50}$
9. $\frac{11}{48}$

Objective 6.9 Skill Sharpener

1. $3\frac{3}{5}$
3. $6\frac{1}{2}$
5. $3\frac{3}{10}$
7. $7\frac{3}{4}$
9. $3\frac{1}{10}$

Objective 6.10 Skill Sharpener

1. $1\frac{1}{2}$
3. $2\frac{1}{12}$
5. $1\frac{3}{5}$
7. $2\frac{1}{3}$
9. $3\frac{3}{16}$

Objective 6.11 Skill Sharpener

1. 1, 2, 4, 8
3. 1, 2, 3, 4, 6, 12
5. 1, 2, 3, 4, 6, 8, 12, 24
7. 1, 2, 5, 10
9. 1, 2, 7, 14

Objective 6.12 Skill Sharpener

1. 1, 2, 4
3. 1, 5
5. 1
7. 1, 3
9. 1, 3

Objective 6.13 Skill Sharpener

1. 3
3. 3
5. 1
7. 1
9. 1

Objective 6.14 Skill Sharpener

1. $\frac{3}{4}$
3. $\frac{1}{9}$
5. $\frac{1}{2}$
7. $\frac{1}{2}$
9. $\frac{1}{2}$

Objective 6.15 Skill Sharpener

1. P
3. I
5. P
7. I
9. P

Objective 6.16 Skill Sharpener

1. P
3. I
5. P
7. P
9. I

Objective 6.17 Skill Sharpener

1. $1\frac{1}{8}$
3. 4
5. $1\frac{1}{2}$
7. 4
9. $6\frac{1}{3}$

Objective 6.18 Skill Sharpener

1. 4, 8, 12, 16, 20, 24, 28, 32, 36, 40. . .
3. 6, 12, 18, 24, 30, 36, 42, 48, 54, 60. . .
5. 8, 16, 24, 32, 40, 48, 56, 64, 72, 80. . .

Objective 6.19 Skill Sharpener

1. 4
3. 20
5. 14
7. 18
9. 36

Objective 6.20 Skill Sharpener

1. 6
3. 16
5. 20
7. 24
9. 60

Objective 6.21 Skill Sharpener

1. $\frac{5}{6}$
3. $1\frac{5}{8}$
5. 1
7. $\frac{5}{16}$
9. $\frac{15}{16}$

Objective 6.22 Skill Sharpener

1. $\frac{5}{12}$
3. $\frac{7}{15}$
5. $\frac{1}{2}$
7. $\frac{1}{6}$
9. $\frac{13}{72}$

Objective 6.23 Skill Sharpener

1. $3\frac{4}{7}$
3. $4\frac{1}{4}$
5. $2\frac{5}{8}$
7. $2\frac{5}{8}$
9. $\frac{39}{40}$

Objective 6.24 Skill Sharpener

1. $\frac{29}{9}$
3. $\frac{11}{4}$
5. $\frac{14}{11}$
7. $\frac{81}{12}$
9. $\frac{126}{10}$

Objective 6.25 Skill Sharpener

1. $\frac{1}{2}$
3. $\frac{7}{10}$
5. $\frac{1}{4}$
7. $\frac{3}{16}$
9. $\frac{7}{90}$

Objective 6.26 Skill Sharpener

1. $\frac{1}{9}$
3. $\frac{1}{4}$
5. $\frac{10}{21}$
7. $\frac{7}{12}$
9. $\frac{1}{15}$

Objective 6.27 Skill Sharpener

1. 8
3. $3\frac{1}{5}$
5. 5
7. 6
9. $2\frac{13}{16}$

Objective 6.28 Skill Sharpener

1. $2\frac{1}{3}$
3. $\frac{7}{10}$
5. 2
7. $\frac{38}{77}$
9. $2\frac{18}{21}$

Objective 6.29 Skill Sharpener

1. $1\frac{1}{2}$
3. $1\frac{5}{27}$
5. 2
7. $6\frac{4}{5}$
9. $4\frac{67}{160}$

CHAPTER 7 RATIOS AND PROPORTIONS

Self-Assessment Pretest

1. 7:8
2. 3:12
3. 33:66
4. 9:27
5. 20:30
6. 3:2
7. 1:3
8. 12:48
9. 24:6
10. 38:3
11. equal
12. not equal
13. not equal
14. not equal
15. equal
16. equal
17. not equal
18. equal
19. not equal
20. not equal
21. x = 3
22. x = 360
23. x = 18
24. x = 270,000
25. x = 2
26. x = 0.7
27. x = 24.5
28. x = 1
29. $x = 330.\overline{66}$
30. x = 86.78996
31. 7.5 mL
32. 3.36%
33. 10 mL
34. 6 mL
35. 20%
36. 83.87%
37. $1\frac{1}{2}$ mL
38. 11.88%
39. yes
40. 0.156 second

Objective 7.3 Skill Sharpener

1. equal
3. equal
5. equal
7. not equal
9. not equal

Objective 7.4 Skill Sharpener

1. x = 24
3. x = 578
5. x = 30,000
7. $x = 7.\overline{33}$
9. x = 129.85074

Objective 7.5 Skill Sharpener

1. 3 mL
3. 2
5. 1 mL
7. $35 per hour
9. 3.9473684%

CHAPTER 8 PERCENTAGES

Self-Assessment Pretest

1. 45%
2. 78%
3. 89%
4. 91%
5. 33.41%
6. 25.56%
7. 87.3%
8. 11.2%
9. 49.4%
10. 100%
11. 0.34
12. 0.57
13. 0.12
14. 0.9
15. 0.43
16. 0.7567
17. 0.3944
18. 0.11901
19. 0.85554
20. 0.2245
21. 262.5
22. 20.145
23. 1,188
24. 29.975
25. 10,511.847
26. 0.06
27. 3.366
28. 11,661
29. 21.44
30. 2.7
31. 45%
32. 25%
33. 13%
34. 72.996479%
35. 14%
36. 32%
37. 3%
38. 12%
39. 1.8%
40. 9%
41. $652.91
42. $1,185.75
43. 104
44. $17.70
45. $30
46. 65%
47. 53.14%
48. $134.06
49. 31 cents
50. 37%

Objective 8.2 Skill Sharpener

1. 37.5%
3. 183.2%
5. 233.23%
7. 4,543.243%
9. 98.23%

Objective 8.3 Skill Sharpener

1. 0.34
3. 0.039
5. 0.75532
7. 0.312594
9. 0.0845

Objective 8.4 Skill Sharpener

1. 262.5
3. 247.5
5. 800
7. 7.5
9. 42.25
11. 33%
13. $6.\overline{66}\%$
15. 25%
17. 18.42105%
19. 64%

Objective 8.5 Skill Sharpener

1. 110.5
3. 40.625
5. 14.592

7. 1.35
9. 63.365
11. 12.5%
13. 22%
15. 52%
17. 7%
19. 97%

CHAPTER 9 CONVERSIONS

Self-Assessment Pretest

1. $\frac{11}{25}$
2. $\frac{17}{25}$
3. $\frac{23}{100}$
4. $\frac{11}{100}$
5. $\frac{49}{50}$
6. $\frac{77}{100}$
7. $\frac{7}{8}$
8. $\frac{17}{50}$
9. $\frac{1}{8}$
10. $\frac{9}{10}$
11. 46%
12. 12.5%
13. 33%
14. 87%
15. 58%
16. 91%
17. 74%
18. 24%
19. 65%
20. 31.2%
21. 0.44
22. 0.9
23. 0.68
24. 0.55
25. 0.8
26. 0.4375
27. $0.\overline{33}$
28. 0.8461538
29. $0.8\overline{18}$
30. 0.68
31. 74.5%
32. 37.5%
33. $6.\overline{66}$%
34. $66.\overline{66}$%
35. $36.\overline{36}$
36. 45%
37. $96.\overline{96}$%
38. 70%
39. 36.8%
40. 65.7%
41. $\frac{17}{50}$
42. $\frac{57}{100}$
43. $\frac{87}{100}$
44. $\frac{33}{50}$
45. $\frac{3}{25}$
46. $\frac{1}{8}$
47. $\frac{77}{100}$
48. $\frac{4}{5}$
49. $\frac{429}{1000}$
50. $\frac{23}{100}$
51. 0.13
52. 0.61
53. 0.59
54. 0.31
55. 0.98
56. 0.5
57. 0.66
58. 0.8
59. 0.34
60. 0.99
61. 3000
62. 1200
63. 1.3
64. 595
65. 240
66. 2
67. 2
68. 3
69. 16
70. 12

Objective 9.1 Skill Sharpener

1. $\frac{19}{50}$
3. $\frac{233}{1000}$
5. $\frac{1}{4}$
7. $\frac{9}{10}$
9. $2\frac{3}{4}$

Objective 9.2 Skill Sharpener

1. 34%
3. 87%
5. 39%
7. 90%
9. 123%

Objective 9.3 Skill Sharpener

1. 0.5
3. 0.8
5. 0.9
7. 0.375
9. $0.\overline{33}$

Objective 9.4 Skill Sharpener

1. 80%
3. 12.5%
5. $33.\overline{33}$%
7. $51.\overline{11}$%
9. 43.75%

Objective 9.5 Skill Sharpener

1. $\frac{23}{100}$
3. $\frac{9}{10}$
5. $\frac{1}{3}$
7. $\frac{3}{5}$
9. $\frac{9}{10}$

Objective 9.6 Skill Sharpener

1. 0.32
3. 0.67
5. 0.03
7. 0.91
9. 0.009

Objective 9.7 Skill Sharpener

1. 0.056
3. 0.034
5. 230
7. 0.029
9. 2300

Objective 9.8 Skill Sharpener

1. 1.07
3. 1
5. 240
7. 8
9. 32

Objective 9.9 Skill Sharpener

1. 1
3. 8
5. 2
7. 2
9. $1\frac{1}{2}$

Objective 9.10 Skill Sharpener

1. 360
3. 720
5. 15
7. $2\frac{1}{2}$
9. 2

CHAPTER 10 MEDICATION DOSAGE CALCULATIONS

Self-Assessment Pretest

1. NDC number
2. Manufacturer
3. Warning
4. Trade name
5. Generic name
6. Usual adult dose
7. Dosage strength
8. Drug form
9. Total amount enclosed
10. Lot number
11. Physician's name
12. Patient's name
13. Refill blank
14. Designation to label
15. Generic substitution allowed
16. Dispense as written
17. Instructions for taking medication
18. Subscription
19. Physician address
20. Patient address
21. $1\frac{1}{2}$ mL
22. 5 mL
23. 2 mL
24. 1 mL
25. 4 mL
26. 1 mL
27. 4 mL
28. 2 mL
29. $\frac{1}{2}$ mL
30. $2\frac{1}{2}$ mL
31. 500 mL
32. 600 mL
33. 200 mL
34. 200 mL
35. 500 mL
36. 300 mL
37. 400 mL
38. 800 mL
39. 700 mL
40. 100 mL
41. 21 gtts/min
42. 25 gtts/min
43. 10 gtts/min
44. 50 gtts/min
45. 33 gtts/min
46. 8 8%
47. 12 12%
48. 25 25%
49. 15 15%
50. 3 3%
51. 0.36 gm
52. 4 gm
53. 2.7 gm
54. 0.2 gm
55. 0.05 gm
56. 3.75 mL
57. 3 mL
58. 7 mL
59. 10 mL
60. 0.6 mL
61. Place one tablet under your tongue as needed for chest pain.
62. Take 3 tablets by mouth three times/day.
63. Take 3 tablets twice a day until gone (7 days).
64. Take 1 teaspoon twice a day.
65. Take 2 teaspoons by mouth twice a day.

Objective 10.1 Skill Sharpener

1. Trade name: Comvax
   Generic name: Haemophilus b Conjugate and Hepatitis B Vaccine
   Manufacturer: Merck and Company
   NDC number: 0006-4898-00
   Dosage strength: 7.5 mcg of Hib, 125 mcg Neisseria meningitides, and 5 mcg of hepatitis B surface antigen
   Drug form: liquid
   Usual adult dose: 0.5 mL
   Amount enclosed: 10 vials
   Prescription warning: not seen
   Expiration date: not seen
   Lot number: not seen
3. Trade name: Mevacor
   Generic name: Lovastatin
   Manufacturer: Merck
   NDC number: 0006-0731-61
   Dosage strength: 20 mg
   Drug form: tablets
   Usual adult dose: not seen
   Amount enclosed: 60
   Prescription warning: not seen
   Expiration date: December 1997
   Lot number: B3143
5. Trade name: Celebrex
   Generic name: celecoxib
   Manufacturer: Pfizer, Searle
   NDC number: 0025-1520-31 (100 mg) 0025-1525-31 (200 mg)
   Dosage strength: 100 mg or 200 mg
   Drug form: tablet
   Usual adult dose: not seen
   Amount enclosed: 100
   Prescription warning: not seen
   Expiration date: not seen
   Lot number: not seen

Objective 10.2 Skill Sharpener

1. Diptheria and tetanus toxoids and acellular pertussis vaccine adsorbed
3. No. It is on the back of the package.
5. not seen
7. Not seen
9. drug form, usual dose, expiration date, lot number

Objective 10.3 Skill Sharpener

1. Lane Kennamer
3. Dora Reid
5. not shown
7. Yes, two.
9. take thou

Objective 10.4 Skill Sharpener

1. 3 mL
3. 8 mL
5. 9 mL

Objective 10.5 Skill Sharpener

1. remaining: 300 mL
   infused: 700 mL
3. remaining: 200 mL
   infused: 800 mL
5. remaining: 100 mL
   infused: 900 mL

Objective 10.6 Skill Sharpener

1. 10 gtts/min
3. 23 gtts/min
5. 50 gtts/min

Objective 10.7 Skill Sharpener

Concentration of solutions

1. 4 4%
3. 50 50%
5. 9 9%

Percent strength

1. 0.6 gm
3. 5.25 gm
5. 1.08 gm

Objective 10.8 Skill Sharpener

1. 48 mL
3. 3.25 mL
5. 3
7. 0.5 mL
9. 0.8 mL

Objective 10.9 Skill Sharpener

1. Take 1 tablespoon of the cough syrup by mouth.
3. Take 1 tablet every 4 hours as needed for nausea.
5. Allow one tablet to dissolve under your tongue as needed for chest pain.
7. Take 2 tablets by mouth twice a day.
9. Take 2 tablespoons of the medication after meals.

CHAPTER 11 WEIGHTS AND MEASURES

Self-Assessment Pretest

1. 195 lb
2. 115 lb
3. 80 lb
4. 48 lb
5. 160 lb
6. 68 kg
7. 101 kg
8. 11 kg
9. 18 kg
10. 75 kg
11. 70 kg
12. 113 kg
13. 5 kg
14. 1 kg
15. 3 kg
16. 150 lb
17. 20 lb
18. 713 lb
19. 165 lb
20. 200 lb
21. 220 lb
22. 26 lb
23. 64 lb
24. 145 lb
25. 282 lb
26. $5\frac{1}{4}''$
27. $2\frac{5}{8}''$
28. $1\frac{3}{8}''$
29. 4″
30. $3\frac{1}{8}''$
31. $6\frac{1}{2}$ cm or 65 mm
32. 110 mm or 11 cm
33. 5 cm or 50 mm
34. 40 mm or 4 cm
35. 82 mm or 8.2 cm
36. 5.18 meters
37. 8.26 meters
38. 182.88 cm
39. 10.16 cm
40. 63.5 mm
41. 193.04 cm
42. 240 cm
43. 441.96 cm
44. 3.81 m
45. 30.18 m
46. 9.84 ft
47. 39.36 ft
48. 108.24 ft
49. 17.7 in
50. 23 in
51. 363.2 in
52. 2.2 in
53. 713.95 yd
54. 278.9 ft
55. 51 in
56. 104°F
57. 95.6°F
58. 101.2°F
59. 100.8°F
60. 98.6°F
61. 103.4°F
62. 96.8°F
63. 101.4°F
64. 99.2°F
65. 98.8°F
66. 37°C
67. 25.6°C
68. 38.9°C
69. 12.8°C
70. 676.7°C
71. 100°C
72. 162.8°C
73. 232.2°C
74. 482.2°C
75. –17.2°C
76. 53.6°F
77. 93.2°F
78. 131°F
79. 71.6°F
80. 244.4°F
81. 253.4°F
82. 453.2°F
83. 194°F
84. 73.4°F
85. 269.6°F
86. 0.68 m^2
87. 0.22 m^2
88. 0.98 m^2
89. 2m^2
90. 0.18 m^2

Objective 11.1 Skill Sharpener

1. 135 lb
3. 148 lb
5. 35 lb

Objective 11.2 Skill Sharpener

1. 100 kg
3. 18 kg
5. 89 kg
7. 41 kg
9. 91 kg
11. 121 lb
13. 242 lb
15. 26 lb
17. 341 lb
19. 275 lb

Objective 11.3 Skill Sharpener

1. $2\frac{1}{2}''$
3. $3\frac{3}{4}''$
5. 2″
7. $1\frac{3}{8}''$
9. $5\frac{1}{4}''$

Objective 11.4 Skill Sharpener

1. 3 cm or 30 mm
3. 79 mm or 7.9 cm
5. 40 mm or 4 cm
7. $11\frac{1}{2}$ cm or 115 mm
9. 19 mm or 1.9 cm

Objective 11.5 Skill Sharpener

1. 3.05 m
3. 2.82 m
5. 19.82 m
7. 13.72 m
9. 5.34 m
11. 62.32 ft
13. 42.64 ft
15. 275.52 ft
17. 181.48 ft
19. 52.48 ft
21. 36″
23. 30″
25. 59.06″
27. 40″
29. 21″

Objective 11.6 Skill Sharpener

1. 99.0°F
3. 99.2°F
5. 98.4°F
7. 98.6°F
9. 99.4°F

Objective 11.7 Skill Sharpener

1. 48.9°C
3. 37.6°C
5. 39.4°C
7. 32.2°C
9. 43.3°C
11. 89.6°F
13. 55.2°F
15. 131°F
17. 73.2°F
19. 62.2°F

Objective 11.8 Skill Sharpener

1. 0.9 m^2
3. 1.34 m^2
5. 1.2 m^2
7. 1.75 m^2
9. 0.27 m^2

CHAPTER 12 MEASURING INTAKE AND OUTPUT

Self-Assessment Pretest

1. 200 mL
2. 150 mL
3. 350 mL
4. 600 mL
5. 400 mL
6. 2,100 mL
7. 2,550 mL
8. 1,800 mL
9. 1,650 mL
10. 2,400 mL
11. 960 mL
12. 740 mL
13. 960 mL
14. 500 mL
15. 850 mL
16. 240 mL
17. 480 mL
18. 65 mL
19. 160 mL
20. 90 mL
21. retained 100 mL
22. retained 20 mL
23. 50 mL more output than intake
24. 145 mL more output than intake
25. retained 50 mL

Objective 12.2 Skill Sharpener

1. 100 mL
3. 210 mL
5. 230 mL
7. 150 mL
9. 310 mL

Objective 12.3 Skill Sharpener

1. 1,800 mL
3. 2,120 mL
5. 1,750 mL
7. 2,145 mL
9. 1,700 mL

Objective 12.4 Skill Sharpener

1. 360 mL
3. 860 mL
5. 1,680 mL

Objective 12.5 Skill Sharpener

1. 50 mL retention
3. balance
5. 2,610 mL

APPENDIX E FINAL SUMMATIVE EVALUATION

1. 144 lb
3. A
5. every 6 hours
7. Lilly
9. 8 mL
11. 60
13. 68°F–77°F
15. 2920 mL
17. 25 gtts/min
19. 20%
21. 3 times a day—breakfast, lunch, dinner
23. 9 tablets
25. 9 mL

INDEX